The Intentional Mentor
in Medicine

The Intentional Mentor in Medicine

A Toolkit for Mentoring Doctors

Dianne Salvador
Dr Joel Wight

Published by Dianne Salvador and Dr Joel Wight
For enquiries, contact toolkit4mentoringdoctors@gmail.com

This book has been prepared and published for educational purposes only. It is not intended as a substitute for legal or other professional advice. While every precaution has been taken in preparation of this book, the publishers and authors assume no responsibility for any errors or omissions, factual or otherwise, or for any losses or damages that you may suffer as a result of the use of information contained in this book. Before relying on the material contained in this book you should carefully evaluate the source, accuracy, currency, completeness and relevance of the information for your purpose. You should seek your own professional and/or legal advice prior to implementing any of the information or processes contained in this book. The publishers and authors shall not be held liable or responsible to any entity with respect to any loss or damages caused, or alleged to have been caused, directly or indirectly arising from the information contained in this book.

The Cambridge Model. From "The relationship between competence and performance: Implications for assessing practice performance", by J. Rethans, et al. (2002). *Medical Education*, 36(10), 901–909. Copyright 2002 by Blackwell Science Ltd. Reproduced with permission.

The CanMEDS Framework. From Frank, J.R., Snell, L., & Sherbino, J. (Eds.) (2015). *CanMEDS 2015 physician competency framework*. Ottawa: Royal College of Physicians and Surgeons of Canada. Reproduced with permission.

Acquisition of performance. From K. A. Ericsson's "The influence of experience and deliberate practice on the development of superior expert performance", In K. A. Ericsson, N. Charness, P. Feltovich, and R. R. Hoffman Eds. *Cambridge handbook of expertise and expert performance* p.695. Copyright 2006 Cambridge University Press. Reproduced with permission.

Design: Zephyrmedia
Indexing: Alpha Indexing
Cover photography: Maddy Voinea
Cover models: Dr Richard Gartrell and Dr Phoebe O'Hare

National Library of Australia
Cataloguing-in-publication entry
Salvador, Dianne, author.
The intentional mentor in medicine: a toolkit for mentoring doctors / Dianne Salvador & Dr Joel Wight.
ISBN: 9780646955216 (paperback)
Includes index.
Mentoring in medicine – Australia.
Physicians – Training of – Australia.
Mentoring in the professions – Australia.
Wight, Joel, author.
610.69507155

Contents

List of illustrations

TABLES

Preface

If you have picked up this book, chances are you are a doctor who is motivated to perform the role of mentor to junior medical colleagues. Perhaps you are already involved in mentoring, offering mentoring on the run during your day to day work, or delivering mentoring within a formal mentoring program. This book is designed to help you to develop as a mentor to junior medical colleagues, and to contribute to developing a mentoring culture in the field of medicine.

We wrote this book because we saw a need. Every doctor is also an educator, but doctors are rarely taught how to educate. Some doctors are naturally gifted educators, and many are invested enough to go one step further and become mentors who guide junior medical colleagues in how to think and learn, and how to develop professional skills, practices, values and identity. Many of you will have been doing this already, without calling it 'mentoring.' However, for a profession that stands or falls on how well we all contribute to passing the profession on to the next generation, our current methods of training the trainer are at best inadequate, and at worst, completely absent.

There is a plethora of information about what we should not be doing, for example the Report to the Royal Australasian College of Surgeons (RACS, 2015). The media covers a new story seemingly every week about what is wrong with medical training. We should not bully. We should not belittle. We should not just expect junior doctors to be able to do everything. These issues will continue to mar our profession until we as a profession are able to change medical culture. It is not enough to tell doctors how *not* to teach. We must instead give a positive alternative. Mentoring is not a panacea of medical training; it has its drawbacks. When done properly, it can be time-consuming and it requires real investment in outcomes of individuals, rather than large groups. However, for those of us who are interested in changing medical culture for the better into the future, mentoring is a positive approach.

Imagine if the next generation of doctors were all trained not only by caring and dedicated supervisors, but also by well-prepared, committed mentors. Our hope is that the next generation will be influenced by a positive model of medical training, and will naturally pass that on to the generation that follows. This is the big picture of mentoring. One doctor mentoring one doctor makes a small difference. Nevertheless, if mentoring becomes part of our day-to-day medical practice, we change medical culture.

Acknowledgements

We would first like to acknowledge Dr Rachel Collings, a co-author of a previous work *Mentoring Doctors* and a contributor to this work. Rachel's commitment to mentoring and the professional development of others is inspirational, and this work would not have been possible without her input.

Dr Thomas Skovholt's Cycle of Caring is the foundation and inspiration for our work. We are grateful for Thomas's permission to incorporate his work with ours.

Paul Welch contributed the content for the feature on metacognition in Appendix C. Paul has presented his work on clinical reasoning and metacognition internationally, and we thank him for his valuable contribution.

We would also like to acknowledge Professor Tarun Sen Gupta, who proved a great encouragement and contributed much wisdom gained from his many years of experience in medical education, and Associate Professor Kerrianne Watt, who contributed outcome evaluation content to Chapter 13.

To our spouses, Alex and Shu-en, thanks for your endless patience with us during the writing process.

Lastly, we could not have written this book were it not for the wonderful mentors we have had over our individual careers. Without question, the most influential training and development we have experienced is through mentoring (although we may not have called it that at the time). You are the inspiration for this book. We cannot name you all, but you know who you are. Thank you.

Dianne Salvador and Joel Wight

Introduction

Patients need good doctors; doctors who "make the practice of scientific medicine humanly relevant" (Rabow, Remen, Parmelee & Inui, 2010, p. 314). It follows that the medical profession needs a way of fostering the development of good doctors, and perpetuating all that is good about the medical profession, including the lineage values of compassion, healing and service. Mentoring is a way to do this.

Some might perceive mentoring as a soft process, inadequate for the rigor of medical training and the resilience required for medical practice. Of course, the irony of the prevailing sink or swim attitude to medical training is that it does nothing to *develop* resilience; it merely leverages a process of natural selection, allowing only those who are already resilient to continue. But mentoring is not a soft process. Mentors are not care bears. Far from it. Mentoring is an active, dynamic and individualised process that offers challenge, support and facilitation when needed, within a trusting partnership. When resilience is an issue, the mentor is there to encourage its development. Mentoring is not an easy process, as it requires time, investment and care. But it is a vital process, and as you will see, one that adds immensely to our current training models.

As a strategy, mentoring can help achieve a diverse range of developmental outcomes important to individual doctors. It can also help address complex issues important to the medical profession as a whole: guiding professional formation, eliminating bullying, discrimination and sexual harassment, and improving the mental health of doctors.

The book has two overarching, linked themes: doctor development, and how to be a mentor who contributes to doctor development. We use the term *doctor development* as shorthand for the doctor acquiring a repertoire of *knowing* (a dynamic knowledge and skills base), *doing* (a set of performance behaviours) and *being* (awareness and practise of values) relevant to their job and or career path. This breadth of development is central to making the practice of scientific medicine humanly relevant.

A premise of the book is that doctor development is influenced by access to support (strengthening resources), challenge (strain-inducing resources) and facilitation (breakthrough-enabling resources), and the mentor can be a contributor of these resources through relational and developmental work. The mentor's relational and development work is performed with ten tools: purposeful communication, partnership, goal-directed interaction, curriculum and performance standards, brief intervention, resilience work, career guidance, confidentiality, evaluation and reflective practice of mentoring.

The book is divided into three parts. Part One is theoretical and begins with the aim of clarifying the mentoring phenomenon, defining mentoring as a purpose-driven partnership and process (or strategy) for development distinct from other medical education strategies. Two mentoring models are introduced, the Model of Intentional Mentoring, and I-Mentor with the Cycle of Caring based on Skovholt's Cycle of Caring (2005), to visually explain intentional mentoring practices and an approach to the mentor's role. After covering mentoring, Part One explains the concept of doctor development, how doctor development occurs, and why development is relevant to all doctors irrespective of seniority. It describes the developmental needs of doctors and four sources of information about developmental needs: felt, expressed, comparative and normative needs, each relevant to developmental work in mentoring. It introduces the three facets of the mentor's role, doing relational work, doing developmental work, and giving structure to mentoring.

Part Two is practical and contains the toolkit of ten tools for mentoring doctors, promised in the subtitle of this book. To produce the desired effects with the tools, skills are required. The toolkit and associated appendices include guidelines for drawing on the required skills to use the tools constructively and productively during mentoring.

Part Three is illustrative and covers mentoring in practice and the application of the tools, through the case of Sam, a general physician and Mikey, a medical registrar. The case study shows the relevance and versatility of the tools, and presents ideas on how to apply the tools in a diverse range of mentoring scenarios.

Figure 1 illustrates the main concepts covered in this book.

Doctor
development
see Chapter 2

Developing a culture of
mentoring in medicine
see Chapter 18

Developmental
needs of doctor
see Chapter 3

Mentoring as
a partnership
see Chapter 1

Intentional mentoring as a
constructive partnership and
productive process for development
*(represented by the Model of
Intentional Mentoring)*
see Chapter 1

Mentoring as a
process for
development
see Chapter 1

An intentional approach
to the mentor's role
*(represented by I–Mentor
with the Cycle of Caring)*
see Chapter 4

Relational work
see Chapter 4

Structuring the partnership and process
see Chapter 4

Developmental work
see Chapter 4

The versatile
mentor
see Chapter 17

The intentional mentor's toolkit

Reflective practice
of mentoring
see Chapter 14

Purposeful
communication
see Chapter 5

Evaluation
see Chapter 13

Partnership
see Chapter 6

Confidentiality
see Chapter 12

Goal-directed
interaction
see Chapter 7

Career guidance
see Chapter 11

Curriculum and
performance standards
see Chapter 8

Resilience work
see Chapter 10

Brief intervention
see Chapter 9

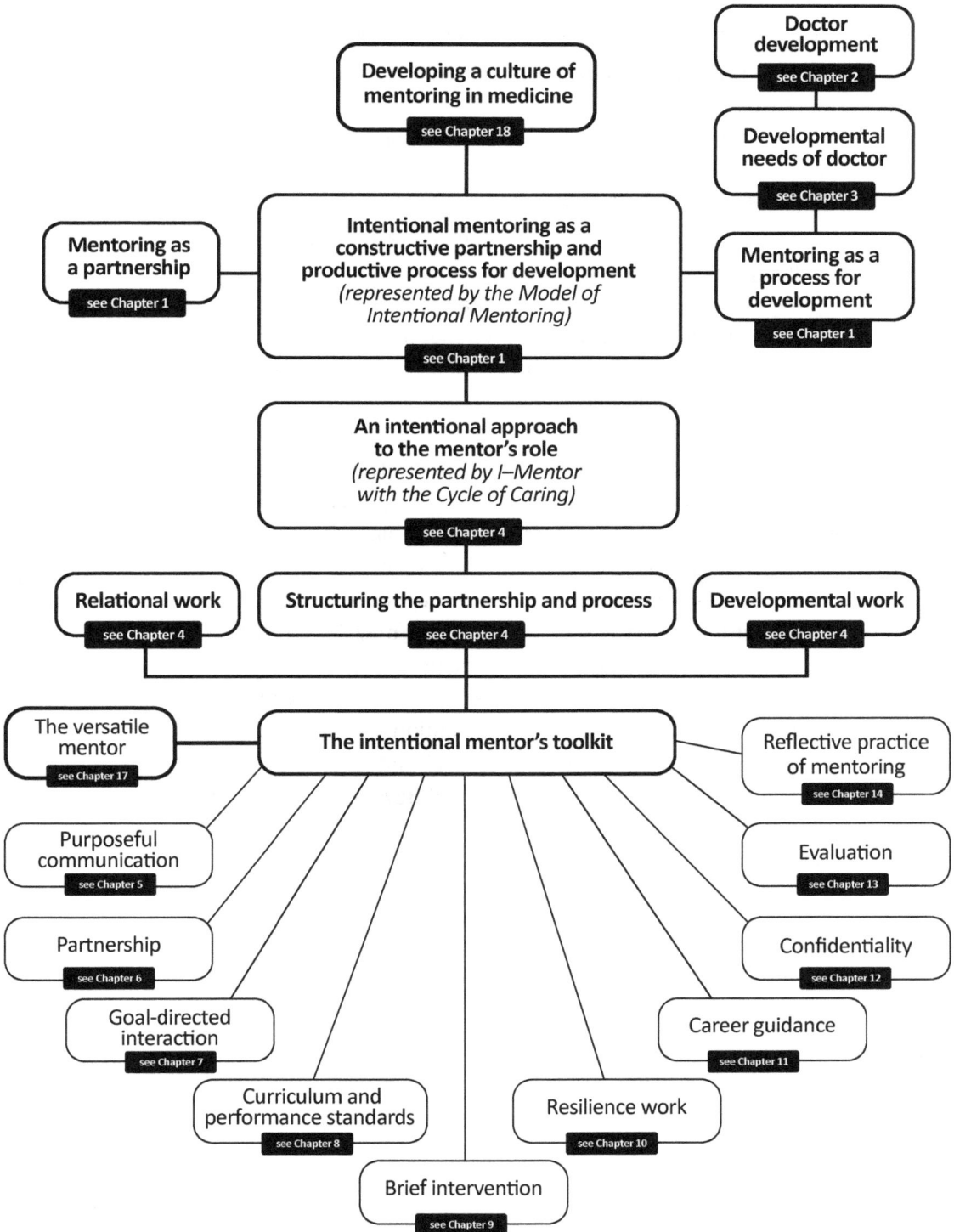

Figure 1. The structure of *The Intentional Mentor in Medicine*

As you read *The Intentional Mentor in Medicine* you will discover how to:

- perform the mentor's portion of the relational and developmental work of mentoring
- add structure to a mentoring partnership and process
- create a safe space for the mentee to access personalised assistance as they pursue developmental outcomes that are meaningful to them
- recognise and respond to the mentee's developmental needs for support, challenge and facilitation
- deliver support, challenge and facilitation in constructive and productive ways
- avoid any form of exploitation of the mentee or harm to the mentee
- apply principles and practices of teaching and giving feedback
- contribute to the mentee's development as a doctor in practice.

The book is designed to be a predominantly practical guide to mentoring with a focus on how to perform the role of mentor. Although theory is a necessary inclusion to provide a foundation for learning the role of mentor, we limit the theoretical component by covering theories in simplified forms applicable to mentoring in the medical profession, and by using tables and figures liberally throughout the book and the appendices. Readers who wish to skip the bulk of the theory may like to start at Part 2, p.59. For readers who want more theory, the References section points to fuller explanations, and the Annotated Bibliography features articles that we highly recommend. As we introduce numerous concepts and definitions, a glossary is provided to clarify terminology. Being a practical guide, this book is not just for reading, it is for actioning. After building your toolkit, your relational and developmental work as an intentional mentor begins.

1

Part One:
Mentoring concepts and theory

1. Intentional mentoring in medicine: A strategy for doctor development

The elusive concept of mentoring

Perspectives on the meaning of mentoring are widely diverse, prompting Bozeman and Feeney to aptly remark "If everything is mentoring, then nothing is" (2007, p.731). Hagerty (1986) suggests that "the literature confuses the person, the process, the purposes and the activities" and "the various authors are describing different phenomena or, at least, different dimensions of a broader theory" (p. 17). To resolve difficulties in the definitional clarity of the word mentor and the action mentoring, Roberts (1999) turns to the origin of the word mentor, Homer's epic poem *Odyssey*. He discovers that Homer's character Mentor does not display qualities corresponding to the contemporary view of a mentor as one who counsels, guides, nurtures and advises. Instead, it is Fénelon's character Mentor in *Les Aventures de Télémaque* who resembles the way we think of a mentor today (Roberts, 1999; 2000; *see also* the Annotated Bibliography section, p.263). Roberts' subsequent review of the literature across decades and disciplines reveals a consensus view of mentoring as having seven essential attributes: a process form, an active relationship, a helping process, a teaching-learning process, reflective practice, a career and personal development process, a formalised process, and a role constructed by or for a mentor (Roberts, 2000).

In the medical profession, definitions of mentoring include:

> "The process whereby an experienced, highly regarded, empathic person (the mentor), guides another individual (the mentee) in the development and re-examination of their own ideas, learning and personal and professional development."
> (Stephen et al., 2008, p.553)

> "Mentoring is an important and productive mechanism for sharing knowledge and expertise between experienced and novice professionals. Mentoring also has the capacity, through dialogic and human relationships, to engender passion and commitment to purpose and cause, and, in so doing, open new directions and opportunities for thought and practice."
> (Australian Public Health Nutrition Academic Collaboration, 2005, p.4)

From these definitions, the idea of mentoring as a process that catalyses transformation of a person, and occurs within and through a partnership of professionals, begins to emerge. Although the definitions are useful for roughly locating mentoring within professional practice, the definitions do not differentiate mentoring from concepts that share similar space such as clinical supervision and teaching, or give specific guidance to either the mentor or the mentee on precisely what to do in mentoring or how to do it. In the medical profession, the delivery of mentoring is structured into doctors' roles, but doctors are seldom given training in mentoring methods and techniques. From our experience, doctors are seeking clarity about the mentoring phenomenon, and appreciate training to perform the mentor role, in order to be effective mentors and fulfil what is recognised as a duty to contribute to the development of succeeding generations of doctors. This chapter aims to clarify the mentoring phenomenon and build foundational knowledge for learning and performing the role of mentor.

Intentional mentoring

What is intentional mentoring?

A partnership and a process for development

Hagerty (1986) provides a revealing clue to solving the definitional difficulties associated with mentoring. She speculates that defining the mentoring phenomenon adequately requires the definition of multiple dimensions and conceptual linkages. Accordingly, our use of the term *intentional mentoring* starts with a view of mentoring as two essential, complementary aspects: a **partnership** and a **process for development**. Separately, neither partnership nor process explains the concept of mentoring, but together they do. This partnership process duality is the essence of mentoring.

The partnership consists of two professionals who:
- have a difference in experience of professional practice
- accept the roles of mentor (the professional with more experience) and mentee (the professional with less experience)
- share an interest in the development of the mentee
- participate voluntarily in the partnership.

The process for development is:

- negotiable, between the mentor and the mentee
- collaborative, with participation by the mentor and the mentee
- interactive, involving exchanges of information and feedback
- goal-oriented, with an emphasis on the mentee's goal setting and achievement
- vision-inspired, informed by an idea of the professional the mentee wants to become.

W.B. Johnson introduces the idea of intentionality in mentoring, suggesting a transition in the mentor's conceptualisation of mentoring (in performing the mentor role), "from secondary or collateral duty to intentional, professional activity" (Johnson, 2002, p.88). Intentional mentoring picks up on Johnson's idea of intentionality. Both the partnership and the process are intentional, not passive. For too long, the medical profession has relied upon doctors' development by osmosis, the idea that "you'll pick it up as you go along." In intentional mentoring, the mentor and the mentee have in mind what they wish to do and achieve.

A mentoring methodology

Intentional mentoring is also a mentoring methodology, a system of principles and practices enacted by the mentor and the mentee during the course of mentoring to enhance the likelihood of mentoring being safe, effective and relevant to the mentee.

Intentional mentoring entails having a **constructive partnership** (relating positively) and using a **productive process for development** (doing more of what works for the mentee's development). Intentional mentoring also involves fulfilling a **purpose** related to the pursuit of developmental outcomes that are meaningful to the mentee.

Three dimensions of the mentee's development are the focus of intentional mentoring – acquiring *knowing* (a dynamic knowledge and skills base), *doing* (a set of performance behaviours) and *being* (awareness and practise of values), each conducive to the mentee adapting and functioning optimally within a particular context. Underpinning the methodology are developmental, learning and socialisation theories that explain transformation (Eby, 2012; Dominguez & Hager, 2013).

Figure 2 depicts intentional mentoring as the pursuit of developmental outcomes that are meaningful to the mentee, at the centre of a constructive partnership and a productive process. The specific principles and practices of intentional mentoring are explored later in this chapter.

Figure 2. Intentional mentoring:
A constructive partnership and
productive process built around
a purpose of development

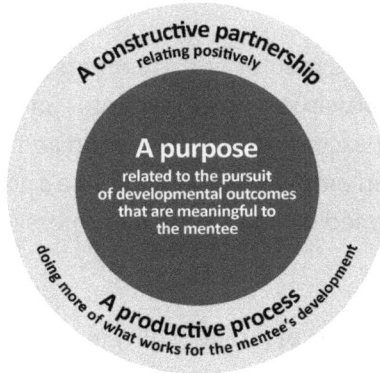

A strategy for doctor development

In this book, we introduce the term *doctor development* as shorthand for the doctor acquiring a repertoire of knowing, doing and being, relevant to their job and or career path, as shown in Figure 3. A *strategy* is an initiative designed to have a particular effect. In the field of medicine, intentional mentoring is a strategy for doctor development.

Figure 3. Doctor development

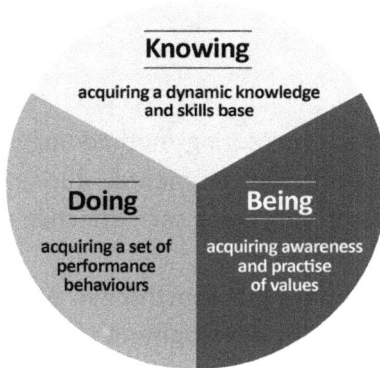

From the perspective of the mentee, the strategy is about developing as a doctor in practice. From the perspective of the mentor, the strategy is about assisting the doctor in practice to develop and adapt. Three types of resources are particularly significant to doctor development – support (strengthening resources), challenge (strain-inducing resources) and facilitation (breakthrough-enabling resources), as you will discover in Chapter 3, pp.35–7.

Ideally, intentional mentoring as a doctor development strategy leads to positive effects on various beneficiaries, including the mentee (e.g. effective functioning in their work context), patients (e.g. good health outcomes and improved personal experiences of health), the mentor (e.g. rewarding experiences and the opportunity to give back to the medical profession), and the medical community (e.g. doctors experiencing collegiality and a collaborative culture). The efforts of two, the mentor and the mentee, are potentially for the benefit of many.

Comparing intentional mentoring and other doctor development strategies

Intentional mentoring is one of a set of strategies for doctor development within clinical training systems. Other notable examples of strategies for doctor development are clinical supervision, teaching and coaching. While these strategies may share similar concept space as mentoring, they are not the same. The aspects of intentional mentoring, partnership and process for development, are useful for revealing distinctions.

Clinical supervision

Like a mentoring partnership, a clinical supervision relationship involves a more experienced and a less experienced doctor. However, the relationship is usually a compulsory line management relationship (or management arrangement devolved from the line manager). A focus of clinical supervision is monitoring and increasing compliance with performance standards. The focus does not necessarily extend to exploring areas of practice that excite the supervisee, or covering topics that the supervisee is passionate about, or assisting the supervisee to achieve ever higher levels of performance. A senior doctor who is performing a mandated clinical supervision role is a clinical supervisor, not a mentor, according to our criteria for mentoring.

Teaching

Many doctors think that if they teach, especially in clinical settings, they are mentoring. However, there is a difference between imparting facts, concepts and principles during teaching, and enabling learning and performance of a craft and profession during mentoring. The focus of teaching is usually on the learner's acquisition of knowledge and skills, and may be based on a generic curriculum. Teaching is frequently delivered in group format and as such, the teacher's relationship with the learner is often in the form of brief engagement.

Coaching

Coaching generally targets certain areas of performance with a view to improving performance. The nature of the partnership tends to be engagement focused on the trainee's performance of specific tasks to a desired level, rather than the trainee's development holistically. The process incorporates exercises in applying particular knowledge and skills, and dealing with specific challenging situations, such as exam preparation and performance.

Intentional mentoring may incorporate clinical supervision, teaching, coaching and much more

Supervision is necessary for monitoring performance, and teaching is indispensable for facilitating learning of knowledge and skills, but mentoring is key to enabling the intelligent application of knowledge and skills at work and holistic development. Guiding a junior medical colleague in how to think, how to learn, and how to develop professional skills, practices, values and identity are at the heart of intentional mentoring. Intentional mentoring bridges the gap between the formal education and management systems and the realities of practising medicine. This is not to say that clinical supervisors, coaches, teachers and mentors fall into completely different spheres in their developmental roles. There is considerable overlap in their activities, and some clinical supervisors, teachers and coaches truly act as mentors, by creating a safe space for the mentee to access individually-relevant assistance.

Table 1 summarises the comparison of prominent doctor development strategies. Although these strategies differ from intentional mentoring in terms of the nature of the partnership and process for development, intentional mentoring may incorporate these strategies.

Table 1. Medical education strategies for doctor development

STRATEGY	PARTNERSHIP	PROCESS FOR DEVELOPMENT
Clinical supervision	Mandatory supervisory relationship	Activities for increasing compliance with performance standards, including performance assessment and provision of feedback
Teaching	Brief engagement, often in group form	Activities for facilitating learning of knowledge and skills
Coaching	Engagement focused on the mentee's performance of specific tasks to a desired level	Activities for applying particular knowledge and skills or dealing with specific challenging situations
Orientation	Brief engagement	Activities for preparing for work settings, providing an introduction to people, processes and places
Assessment	Brief engagement	Activities for ascertaining the level of competence or performance, to inform future learning and or to determine an achievement result

Principles and practices of intentional mentoring

This section provides an overview of the principles and practices enacted by both the mentor and the mentee during the course of intentional mentoring. The idea of the principles and practices is to enhance the likelihood of mentoring being safe, effective and relevant to the mentee. In chapters 4 to 14, coverage of the principles and practices continues, with a focus on the mentor's role, contributions and tools.

Guiding principles

Intentional mentoring has two foundational, guiding principles that apply in the pursuit of developmental outcomes that are meaningful to the mentee:

- Constructiveness; relate positively.
- Productivity; do more of what works for the mentee's development in ways that are relevant to their job, career path and aspirations in the medical profession.

These two principles guide the work of intentional mentoring: relational work and developmental work.

Relational work

The partnership aspect of mentoring translates to the *relational work* of the mentor and mentee. This is the work that builds relationship between two doctors with a difference in experience, who accept the roles of mentor and mentee, and decide to collaborate for the development of the mentee. Relational work includes building trust, sharing an understanding of the purpose of mentoring and each other's role and responsibilities, fulfilling commitments, and adjusting the partnership as the mentee progresses or as circumstances change. The mentee performs their role as doctor. The mentor, a doctor, does not deliver medical care within the mentoring partnership.

Developmental work

The process aspect of mentoring translates to the *developmental work* of the mentor and the mentee; the work that fosters the mentee's development as a doctor. Developmental work includes activities that are conversation-based (e.g. discussing experiences, options and decisions) and action-based (e.g. demonstrating and practising procedural skills), and noticing and doing more of what works for the mentee's development.

The mentee's aspirational state of development is central to the developmental work. Building on the definition of doctor development, we define *aspirational state of development* as a projection of development; an ideal repertoire of *knowing* (a dynamic knowledge and skills base), *doing* (a set of performance behaviours) and *being* (awareness and practise of values) relevant to the mentee's job, career path and aspirations in the medical profession. Simply put, the mentee's aspirational state of development is an image of the doctor they wish to become. By defining an aspirational state of development, the mentee has a starting point for deriving meaningful and relevant goals for mentoring, as well as goal posts to aim for in developmental work and a benchmark for recognising development.

Aspects of the mentee's aspirational state of development may be mandated as part of a structured training program or registration standard (applicable to all doctors and irrespective of individual interests), for example, safe prescribing, recognition and management of the deteriorating patient, basic life support, evidence-based practice and how to function as part of a team. Other aspects of the mentee's aspirational state of development may be their own choice, based on their interests and passions. Examples include specialist and sub-specialist training, involvement in research, drug development, or public health and policy development. One of the roles of the mentor is to help refine the mentee's awareness of their aspirational state of development. (*see* Appendix K, p.244 for examples).

Though relatively stable, the mentee's aspirational state of development is not static. It is likely to change over time, as the mentee achieves their goals, changes practice settings, or gains clarity about the doctor they wish to become. For example, a junior doctor may not be aware how strongly they value social justice and equitable distribution of resources until they are faced with situations where they are asked to deliver a futile treatment. It may take several encounters with these situations to become aware of their most cherished values.

After the mentee identifies their aspirational state of development, they set and pursue meaningful and relevant goals. Goals that are achieved bring them closer to their aspirational state of development, as depicted in Figure 4. Goals may relate to knowing (e.g. learning goals, for acquiring knowledge and skills), doing (e.g. performance goals, for participating and overcoming barriers to performance), and being (e.g. values-related goals, for recognising and enacting values in practice). The mentor and mentee participate in goal-directed interactions and pay attention to results, discovering and doing more of what works for the mentee's development.

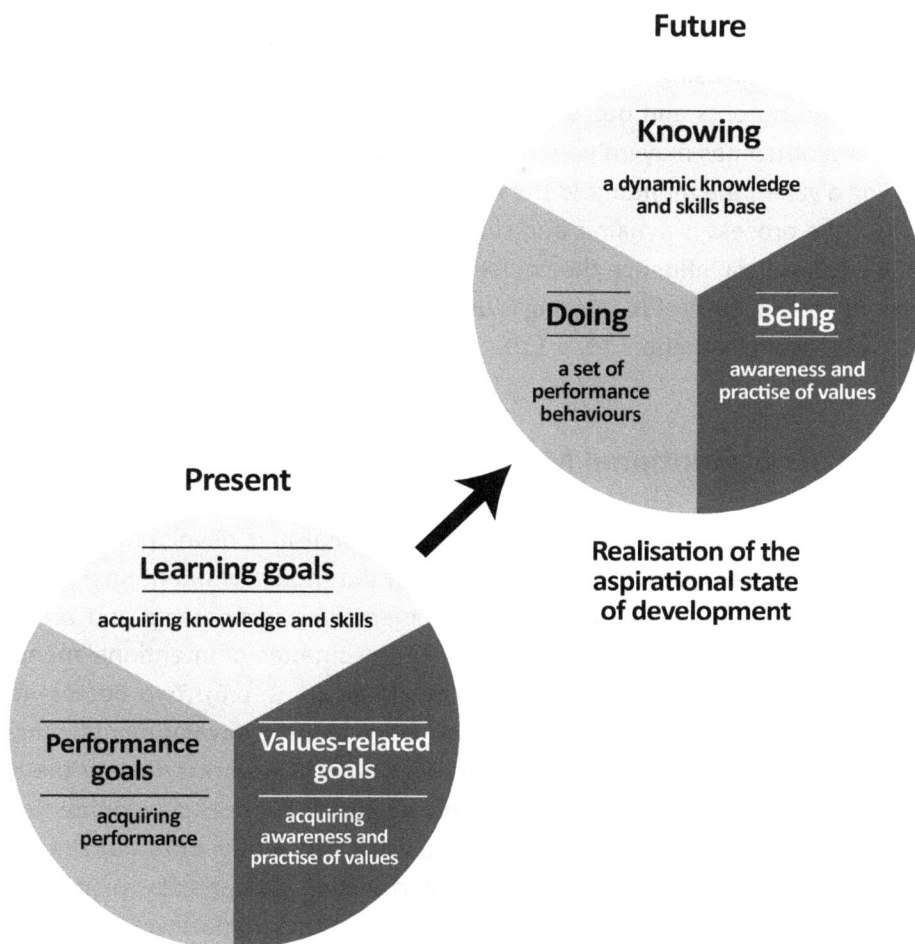

Future

Knowing
a dynamic knowledge
and skills base

Doing
a set of
performance
behaviours

Being
awareness and
practise of values

Present

Learning goals
acquiring knowledge and skills

Performance goals
acquiring
performance

Values-related goals
acquiring
awareness and
practise of values

Realisation of the
aspirational state
of development

Figure 4. Moving towards or realising the aspirational state of development

Transformation

Mentoring catalyses transformation, and being able to recognise transformation (in order to do more of what works for the mentee's development) is part of intentional mentoring. A logic model built from inputs, activities, outputs and outcomes provides a perspective of mentoring that reveals transformation as a sequence of change (MacDonald et al., 2001; Centers for Disease Control and Prevention (CDC), 2008). *Inputs* are the resources invested and used, such as the mentor's and mentee's time and materials. *Activities* are how the inputs are converted into actions in mentoring, for example, mentoring conversations. *Outputs* are the products of mentoring, usually described in numerical terms, including the quantity of activities. Finally, *outcomes* are the intended and unintended results, such as the mentee's goal achievement. However, mentoring is not like using a vending machine; inputs and activities do not always lead to the desired outputs and outcomes, and the transformation is not always linear – outputs and outcomes may influence further inputs and activities. Mentoring is more like sailing a yacht; the mentor and the mentee use the sails to get to where they want to go, but the process is dynamic and subject to other influences – the wind, the tide and the swell will all influence the course they take to arrive at their destination. The logic model perspective of mentoring is useful for evaluation of intentional mentoring and appears again in Chapter 13, p.119.

The Model of Intentional Mentoring

Intentional mentoring practices, that is the relational and developmental work of the mentor and the mentee, are illustrated with the Model of Intentional Mentoring shown in Figure 5. The model represents a mentoring partnership and process of development occurring over time (a dynamic representation of intentional mentoring, in contrast to the static representation shown in Figure 2, p.6). Two doctors form a partnership, do relational and developmental work, achieve developmental outcomes that are meaningful to the mentee, and part ways when the work is done or the time is right. It is cyclical because of feedback: relational work influences developmental work and developmental work influences relational work. The model does not specify how the partnership forms, the duration of the partnership and process, or the number of mentoring sessions. The mentor and the mentee may undertake many cycles of relational work, developmental work, and re-negotiation of the partnership during the course of mentoring. Applications of the model are explained at the end of this chapter, and the model re-appears in Chapter 4, pp.51–4 as the basis of an approach to the mentor's role.

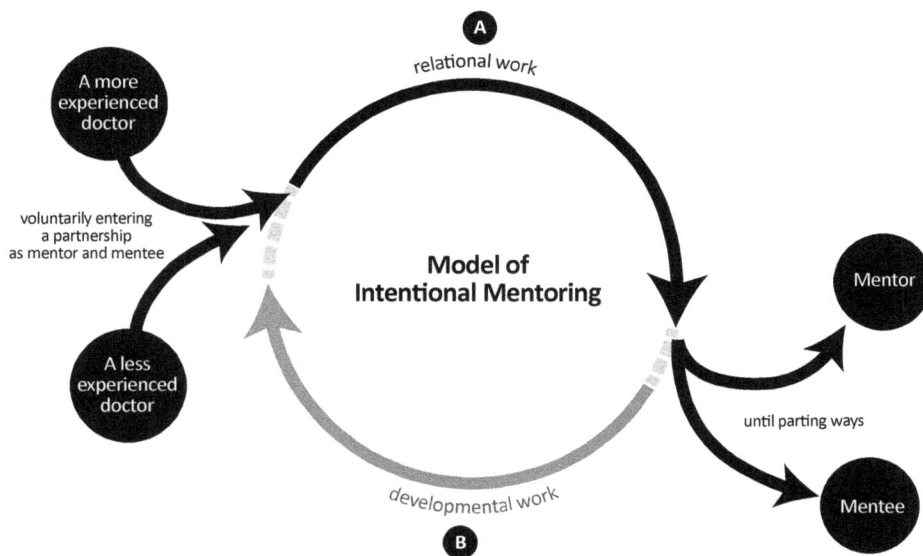

A ASSUMPTIONS

Relational work is work to build relationship

The mentee is a practicing doctor

The mentor is a practicing mentor (not a doctor of the mentee)

They share an interest in the mentee's development as a doctor in practice

They agree to collaborate

The relational work influences the developmental work, and vice versa

B ASSUMPTIONS

Developmental work is work to foster development

The mentee forms an idea of their aspirational state of development

An aspirational state of development is an ideal repertoire of knowing, doing and being

The work involves noticing and doing more of what works for the mentee's development

The work moves the mentee closer to their aspirational state of development

The developmental work influences the relational work, and vice versa

Figure 5. The Model of Intentional Mentoring

Why is intentional mentoring useful in the field of medicine?

Accessing individually-relevant assistance

Intentional mentoring is compatible with clinical training systems that outline a pathway of experiences and milestones for the doctor to pursue towards an advanced state of development. From the mentee's perspective, intentional mentoring offers a safe space to access individually-relevant assistance while pursuing developmental outcomes that are meaningful to them, for example:

- adaptation to the demands of a new job and or work setting
- connectedness and a sense of belonging within the medical community

- socialisation, internalising and abiding by the rules of a group
- awareness of resources for practice
- role clarity
- acquisition of knowledge and skills
- performance improvement
- insight
- helpful habits e.g. being organised
- professionalism
- awareness of values
- resolution of value conflicts
- alleviation of performance anxiety and building and maintaining confidence
- resilience and the capacity to deal effectively with problems
- career path decisions
- readiness for exams.

At the level of the doctor population, intentional mentoring assists all doctors to find solutions to complex issues within the medical profession, such as:

- adapting to change within healthcare organisations
- professional formation
- eliminating bullying, discrimination and sexual harassment
- improving the mental health of doctors.

Adapting to change within healthcare organisations

A healthcare organisation is a complex adaptive system; it is *complex* with diverse agents (e.g. patients and families, clinicians and administrators), *adaptive* with a capacity to change, and a *system* with a set of interconnected agents. The system cannot be decomposed to elements, understood in terms of parts and recomposed into an overall design in the way a traditional system can. A complex adaptive system features five characteristics that highlight and explain change and uncertainty within the system, described in Table 2: learning, nonlinear relationships, self-organisation, emergence and co-evolution (McDaniel, Lanham & Anderson, 2009).

Both medical and mentoring practice are embedded in the complex adaptive system of healthcare organisations. Within the system, work is inseparable from its context (e.g. contextual demands determine aspects of the work to be done) and change is constant (e.g. changes occur in patient expectations, medical knowledge and technology, and perspectives of best practice). There are implications for all participants, with examples shown in Table 2. A significant implication for doctors is that they must continue to develop, adapt and keep up with changes happening around them in order to function optimally at work.

Viewing a healthcare organisation as a complex adaptive system highlights the importance of intentional mentoring as a strategy for developing and adapting within a dynamic healthcare organisation. Through intentional mentoring doctors have the opportunity to share experiences, discover resources, recognise and solve problems, collaborate, innovate, adapt with agility, and find a sense of stability and continuity amidst constant change and uncertainty.

Table 2. Healthcare organisations as complex adaptive systems: implications for medical and mentoring practice

COMPLEX ADAPTIVE SYSTEM CHARACTERISTIC	IMPLICATIONS FOR MEDICAL AND MENTORING PRACTICE
1. Learning Agents operate from their own rules or knowledge, gain experience, learn, and adapt to accommodate the behaviour of other agents	Medical knowledge, methods and systems are continually updated and ongoing learning is required Knowledge is transmitted through both formal curriculum (the stated, endorsed curriculum) and the informal or 'hidden' curriculum (influences on learning operating at the level of the organisation and culture, frequently in interpersonal form)
2. Nonlinear relationships Agents interact and affect each other; cause and effect relationships among agents are not unidirectional and the size of inputs and outputs may be disproportional	Change and uncertainty are ever present Problems often emerge when agents interact due to conflicting values, goals, agenda and behaviours Some problems and solutions can be anticipated and some cannot be anticipated
3. Self-organisation In response to learning and nonlinear relationships, self-organisation occurs and relatively stable patterns of behaviour emerge	Work areas develop ways of doing work or using resources, specific to that area Commencement in a work setting or role requires a time of adaptation and transition
4. Emergence New properties of the system or phenomena appear due to the self-organising behaviour of the system	Innovative solutions emerge, including new products e.g. pharmaceuticals, technologies, treatments and medical devices Priorities emerge, for example, evidence-based healthcare and person-centred care New problems emerge
5. Co-evolution The system evolves with its environment and vice versa	The healthcare organisation evolves with related systems (e.g. government agencies, pharmaceutical companies, and academia) and changes filter through to work areas

Professional formation

A medical practitioner's professional formation involves more than the acquisition of clinical skills and knowledge; professional qualities are also essential. Hafferty and Franks (1994) describe scientific and clinical work as "a fundamentally value-laden enterprise" (p.868). Science offers doctors a range of choices in determining action for patients' care, and a doctor's values guide the application of science. Together, science and values underpin medical decisions.

> "An essential element of medicine's claim to professional status lies in the development of what might be termed a "professional self" in students – the internalization of the values and virtues of medicine as a discipline and a calling. It is not sufficient for students to acquire the knowledge, skills, and outward behavior necessary for practicing medicine. Being a physician – taking on the identity of a true medical professional – also involves a number of value orientations, including a general commitment not only to learning and excellence of skills but also to behavior and practices that are authentically caring…It is this underpinning that provides the necessary stability and generalizability when one has to step outside the realm of textbook medical practice and confront situations of uncertainty and ambiguity – which are, after all, the defining characteristics of real-world medical work."
> (Hafferty, 2006, p. 2152)

Values are variously described as "standards or principles considered valuable or important in life" (Turner & Turner, 1989, p. 895), standards for conduct used as measures of the quality of behaviour, and principles that guide action in daily life. In medicine, ethical values are perhaps the most familiar values to doctors. The four prima facie ethical values, or principles of medical ethics, are beneficence (do good), non-maleficence (do no harm), patient autonomy (respect for patient choice), and justice (fair and equal treatment) (Souba, 2011). Other categories of values described in the literature are science and humanistic values, important for guiding the practice of scientific medicine that is humanly relevant (Rabow, Remen, Parmelee & Inui, 2010). The literature is also replete with articles about professionalism and values associated with professionalism. *Professionalism* is defined as "the norms for the relationships in which physicians engage in the care of patients" (Leach, 2004, p.11) and "a set of values, behaviours, and relationships that underpins the trust that the public has in doctors" (Royal College of Physicians of London, 2005, xi), and encompasses relationships of doctor-patient, doctor-colleagues and profession-society. Professionalism values are important for guiding actions that build trust.

Value conflicts occur when guiding principles differ in decision making, also known as values incongruence (Gabel, 2011). In training and clinical settings many different values are at play and at stake in determining "the best means toward the best ends for individual patients" (Leach, 2004, p. 11). This can be seen in everyday situations in medicine – elective surgery may do good (beneficence) but it may also cause harm (at stake is non-maleficence) through surgical complications. Managing the expense of treatment in a public system with finite resources is a balance between patient autonomy (respect for patient choice) and justice (fair distribution of resources). Conflicts may occur within the doctor (e.g. incongruent personal or cultural and professional values), within the healthcare partnership (e.g. between doctor and patient) and within groups (e.g. the multidisciplinary team and across specialties) and may contribute to 'moral strain', demoralization and burnout (Gabel, 2011).

Values-inconsistent action occurs when values and action are at odds, also described as dissonance between values and practice. The inconsistency may be between the professed and lived values at the cultural level (e.g. the formal curriculum versus the informal curriculum), and may create experiences of 'moral confrontation' for the doctor (Rabow et al., 2010). It may also be inconsistency between professed and lived values at the individual level, when the doctor is not living their authentic values.

Key skills of medical practice are navigating value conflicts, including being able to discern appropriate action in the context of competing values, and aligning values with actions. The training that helps with this is professional formation. Rabow et al. (2010) describe a goal of professional formation: "to tether or anchor students to their personal principles and the core values of the profession" (p.311). Engaging the mentee in professional formation work improves their awareness and practise of values, and is an opportunity for gains such as:

- understanding what motivates behaviour and choices
- discerning the many values at play and at stake in clinical encounters
- integrating personal and professional values
- balancing science and humanistic values
- recognising values-inconsistent actions and triggers
- better alignment of values and actions
- insight through receiving values-focused feedback (*see* Appendix H, p.224).

Intentional mentoring is the ideal context for these activities, providing a space that welcomes the mentee to undertake this highly personal work. The partnership is designed through negotiation to feel safe and comfortable for the mentee and mentor, and the partnership duration can continue for an extended time if needed. In this book, values awareness and practise is a recurring theme, with the doctor development dimension of 'being' devoted to awareness and practise of values.

Eliminating bullying, discrimination and sexual harassment

Bullying is defined by Safe Work Australia as the "repeated and unreasonable behaviour directed towards a worker or a group of workers that creates a risk to health and safety" (http://www.safeworkaustralia.gov.au). Bullying may appear in many forms in the field of medicine, for example 'teaching by humiliation'. In a study by Scott, Caldwell, Barnes and Barrett (2015), 74% of students experienced, and 83.6% witnessed this at the final, clinical-based stage of their degree. Anecdotally, discrimination and sexual harassment may also be present in workplaces where there is a culture of bullying. Due to the power imbalance inherent in hierarchical training, these behaviours are most often directed from senior to junior doctors. Other examples reported in the literature include belittlement (Rautio et al., 2005), mocking and scorn (Phillips & Clarke, 2012) and intimidation/demeaning behaviour (Leape, Shore & Dienstag, 2013). These behaviours reveal a lack of respect for junior medical colleagues and also a lack of concern (or misguided concern) for their welfare and development.

Troublingly, trainees acknowledge and justify the occurrence of intimidation and harassment, using three dimensions of rationalisation: an acceptable purpose attributed to the perpetrator, a positive pedagogical or clinical effect of the behaviour, and a perceived necessity for the behaviour to achieve the purpose (Musselman, MacRae, Reznick & Lingard, 2005). These are hallmarks of behaviour which is engrained in the culture of medicine and which will be perpetuated until the cycle is broken.

In Australia, the problem of bullying, discrimination and sexual harassment reached a crisis point in 2015. Research commissioned by the Expert Advisory Group advising the Royal Australasian College of Surgeons (RACS) found that in surgical specialties, forty-nine percent of fellows, trainees and international medical graduates had been subjected to discrimination, bullying or sexual harassment. The problem was found to exist across all surgical specialities, and senior surgeons and surgical consultants were reported as the primary source of these problems (RACS, 2015). The President of the Royal Australasian College of Surgeons, Professor David Watters OBE, issued an apology on behalf of all fellows, trainees and international medical graduates.

The Expert Advisory Group noted:

> "The status quo will not serve the future. Individually and collectively, College Fellows must recognise and commit to closing the gap between how it has been, and how it must become."
>
> (Royal Australasian College of Surgeons, 2015, p.3)

The recommendations of the Expert Advisory Group revolve around "taking what is best from the rich history of practice and re-settling it on foundations of respect, transparency and professional excellence" (RACS, 2015, p.3). The RACS should be applauded for this response, and we should acknowledge the excellent work done thus far to combat bullying. We also need to acknowledge that the problem is far broader in medical training than just surgery, and that there is still much work to be done.

To illustrate, we will relate the story of a doctor we know. For the sake of confidentiality both the specialty and the name we will use (Sarah) have been changed. Sarah is a hard-working, conscientious young doctor in a procedural training program. She has a gentle and quiet personality and has always performed her studies to a high standard. During the first year of her training, her general thoroughness and attention to detail (qualities previously seen as laudable) meant that procedurally she was slower than her colleagues. Rather than address this directly with a plan to improve her performance, her theatre time was cut back dramatically and she was repeatedly subjected to demeaning language and behaviour at work. This resulted in her falling further behind her colleagues, and developing significant anxiety and depressive features. After many months, a nurse noticed the bullying and intervened on her behalf, and mediation began. However, irreparable damage had been done to the workplace relationships, and Sarah sought to leave her hometown and training hospital, uprooting her life and moving interstate to escape what had become an unworkable situation.

Even today, everyone who has worked in a hospital knows someone like Sarah. What more can be done to solve this problem? A culture of mentoring can be part of the solution. Intentional mentoring is the opposite of bullying. A bully sets an intention to have a negative effect within a relationship. An intentional mentor sets an intention to have a positive effect within a relationship.

There are two main ways that intentional mentoring can help solve the problem of bullying. Firstly, intentional mentoring provides a safe space for the mentee to talk about behaviours that may constitute bullying. The mentee who is bullied may not realise or be able to put a name to the behaviour that is occurring. The mentor can help clarify that the behaviour is in fact inappropriate and constitutes bullying, and also guide the mentee through an appropriate course of action to address the bullying. If Sarah had a mentor, this destructive cycle could have been addressed many months earlier, and the cycle may have been stopped before the damage was irreparable.

Secondly, mentoring on a broader scale at the level of the organisation contributes to cultural change, educating junior doctors through encouragement, care and attention, not through fear or intimidation. If those entrusted with the development of junior doctors acted as mentors rather than bullies, this problem would soon be a thing of the past. If Sarah's supervisors had acted as mentors, helping to address her needs with a constructive plan, this situation could have been avoided entirely.

Improving the mental health of doctors

In 2013, 12,252 doctors and 1,811 medical students responded to The National Mental Health Survey of Doctors and Medical Students, conducted by *beyondblue* (*beyondblue*, 2013). The aims of the survey were to understand and raise awareness of issues associated with the mental health of Australian doctors and medical students, and to guide development and delivery of support services for the medical profession. The survey findings revealed many issues associated with the mental health of doctors, including very high psychological distress, depression, anxiety, suicidal ideation, attempted suicide, work stressors, burnout, stigmatising attitudes and resilience. The survey found that doctors suffer from greater levels of very high psychological distress, depression and suicidal ideation than the general Australian population and other Australian professionals. For junior doctors aged 30 years and under, the level of very high psychological distress was more than ten times higher than for other Australian professionals aged 30 years and under.

Intentional mentoring offers a safe space for mentees to explore how their work is impacting on them, how they are coping and how they stay strong, physically, emotionally, mentally and spiritually. It also offers access to individually-relevant assistance from a mentor who understands the local context and demands, provides 'off the radar' feedback, and can identify developing mental health issues and facilitate professional help as required.

Applications of the Model of Intentional Mentoring in the field of medicine

An approach to mentoring roles

The Model of Intentional Mentoring (*see* Figure 5, p.13) has utility as an approach to the mentor and the mentee roles. Adapting the model to inform the mentor role is described in Chapter 4, pp.51–3 and is central to this book.

An approach to pursuing developmental outcomes

The model indicates how the mentor and mentee can target certain areas of the mentee's practice and collaboratively pursue developmental outcomes that are meaningful to the mentee, such as those listed on pp.13–14.

An approach to planning mentoring

The model provides a perspective of mentoring that can be shared by stakeholders within health organisations, including the mentor, mentee, administrators and policy-makers. With a shared perspective, stakeholders can explore and identify:

- potential costs and benefits of mentoring
- a clear purpose for mentoring
- desired outcomes
- activities likely to lead to the desired outcomes
- the investment or resourcing likely to be required
- roles for stakeholders.

Chapter 18, p.183 presents the application of the model on a large scale as a strategy for expanding the volume of participants in mentoring within a health organisation, and developing a culture of mentoring in the field of medicine.

An approach to mentoring education

The model can also guide mentoring education activities, such as mentor training. By providing an image of mentoring in action and language for explaining mentoring, it makes mentoring amenable to discussion, teaching and learning.

2. Developing as a doctor in practice

Scenario

Mikey led his registrar and resident around the Coronary Care Unit on their usual morning ward round. It was not the most exciting day; only two new patients from the previous evening, one with a non-ST elevation myocardial infarction, and the other with recurrent supraventricular tachycardia. Fairly routine. No surprises.

As they moved from one room to the next, Mikey wondered at what point in time these things became routine, unsurprising. Still enjoyable, of course. Still a source of job satisfaction. But commonplace. Realistically, it was an imperceptible shift over many years. He had been a consultant cardiologist for 3 years now. He was originally interested in neurology, but had changed his mind after having an excellent experience on a cardiology rotation. He was happy with his decision; he loved his job, and he found it very satisfying. It was a good mix for him, with both procedural and non-procedural aspects. He liked emergencies, and quick thinking.

The high pitched wail of the cardiac arrest alarm, triggered by a patient's cardiac telemetry, pierced the air and interrupted Mikey's thoughts. He looked up quickly to see which patient had the issue. Bed 2. Mr Baker. The new patient from last night with a non-STEMI. He saw the nurse rush into the room with the crash trolley. Mikey led the medical team in after them.

As the consultant on the round, he assumed the leadership position. He quickly assessed the situation, and started giving orders.

'Lucy,' he said to his Registrar. 'Take the airway please. Toby,' to his Resident, 'start chest compressions. Jennifer,' the patient's nurse, 'get the pads on as quickly as possible. David,' to the Nurse Unit Manager, who had come to help, 'please call the code and then scribe for us.'

It went on like this. Shock. CPR. Still in VF. Shock again. Another cycle of CPR. Still in VF. Change the person on the chest. Give the adrenaline. Give the amiodarone. More shocks. More chest compressions.

It was a well-run code. The communication was clear. Everything was done correctly. Mikey was good at it. It didn't stress him out much anymore. He just took a deep breath and got on with it.

Unfortunately, as it happens more often than not, it didn't work. After twenty full minutes without spontaneous circulation, Mikey called it.

After a few minutes, he went to tell Mrs Baker. She had been taken to the family room. She was distraught, and Mikey comforted her. He explained, honesty and truly, that they did everything they could. He left her there with one of the hospital social workers for support, and went back out to join his team. They looked equally distraught.

'Let's go have a coffee,' he suggested. They nodded silently, and followed to the CCU staff room. It was empty until they arrived.

'I don't get it,' said Lucy. She was obviously taking it hard; she had admitted the patient the night before. 'What did I miss? I thought we did everything right!'

'We did. You did. What just happened didn't have anything to do with mismanagement or misdiagnosis. Just plain old bad luck. Sometimes we win, and sometimes we don't,' Mikey consoled.

'Before I left last night, he asked me if he was going to be okay. I told him 'Yes, don't worry, you'll be fine. You're in the right place.' How can it go so badly? It was just a small non-STEMI! He should have been fine,' Lucy exclaimed.

Mikey thought for a moment. He thought in particular about a very similar moment in his training, when a young patient had died unexpectedly from a pulmonary embolism. He beat himself up about it for days, until he'd managed to speak to his mentor Sam about it. He had learned a lot since then.

"So what happens now?" Lucy asked.

"Well, any unexpected death in the hospital undergoes review. We will discuss it in our morbidity and mortality meeting, and see if we have missed anything that might have made a difference. That will include a review of all of our performances and the systemic factors that may have contributed."

Lucy recoiled slightly and a worried look furrowed her brow, wondering if she had done anything wrong.

'Lucy,' he said in a comforting tone, 'This is not the last time something like this is going to happen. Losing a patient that you shouldn't have lost always hits you hard. But try and remember two things from this. Firstly, you did everything right, and for the record, you did. I read your admission note. I looked at the drug chart and all the notes. Of course we'll review it all, but from what I can see he was treated appropriately. You need to believe that, because the second thing I want you to remember is this: all we can do is our best. Beyond that, everything is in the lap of the gods.'

They went on talking for a while longer. She will be okay, Mikey thought. It's an awful experience, and one he remembered well. But as he reflected on his own experiences, he was struck by how far he had come since he was a junior registrar. He remembered talking with Sam, setting goals. One of those goals was how to run a code! He obviously had that covered – it was second nature now. But then there were the other things, the other ways Sam had helped him. He had become more resilient. More professional. Much better at clinical reasoning.

All the things that he once thought were daunting, insurmountable tasks he now did with barely a second thought. Thanks, Sam, he thought. Then he got up and went back to the ward round.

> In the scenario, Mikey is working as a consultant cardiologist in the setting of a Coronary Care Unit. The work he does requires him to embody many roles (such as medical expert, leader and communicator), perform at an advanced level and at the highest level of seniority, adapt and respond appropriately to routine and emergent situations, and follow procedures and regulations designed to maximise the safety of his patients. His clinical training years had a focus on learning knowledge and skills, applying his knowledge and skills in the care of diverse patients, and strengthening his awareness of and commitment to values as a foundation for medical practice. Many educators, assessors, supervisors and mentors influenced his development. One mentor, Sam, had a particularly significant influence on his development. *See* Chapter 16, p.139 which explores Sam's work with Mikey.

The scenario was chosen as an illustration of the work of a doctor because it encompasses more than just knowing what to do and how to do it in the practice of scientific medicine – it also takes into account the more humanistic elements of practice such as responding to grief and loss, having a realistic understanding of the limitations of medicine, and building and sustaining resilience. Developing as a doctor in practice involves developing in these areas, and more, in order to function effectively.

This chapter delves into the work of a doctor in practice to find reference points for the developmental work of intentional mentoring. It aims to encourage you to start thinking about what you might help the mentee to develop (e.g. knowledge, skills, performance, and awareness and practise of values), and become (e.g. a doctor who is resourceful, resilient and effective), over the course of mentoring. While recognising that each mentee is unique and developmental work is tailored to the individual, the chapter offers ideas about the content of your developmental work with the mentee.

The work of a doctor in practice

In a book about assisting a mentee to develop as a doctor, the question of what it means to be a doctor, is unavoidable. Godlee (2008) points out that coming up with a definition of what it means to be a doctor is fraught with difficulties because it depends on context, clinical setting, patient preferences, and the doctor's experience and seniority. The Consensus Statement on the Role of a Doctor (http://www.medschools. ac.uk), offers the following definition of a medical doctor.

> "Doctors as clinical scientists apply the principles and procedures of medicine
> to prevent, diagnose, care for and treat patients with illness, disease and
> injury and to maintain physical and mental health. They supervise the
> implementation of care and treatment plans by others in the health care team
> and conduct medical education and research." (p. 1)

Within the statement is an acknowledgment that the role of the doctor is, and will continue to, change with the changing needs and expectations of patients and the development of other healthcare professions. For the purpose of intentional mentoring, and finding enduring reference points for developmental work, we propose four themes in the work of a doctor in practice that are broadly applicable to all doctor jobs in the medical profession.

The four themes relate to performance:

- of roles for meeting the healthcare needs of patients served,
- to the required level of performance of essential tasks,
- in a manner appropriate to the setting, and
- in accordance with regulations.

Performance of roles for meeting the healthcare needs of patients served

The Royal College of Physicians and Surgeons of Canada developed the CanMEDS Framework to articulate a definition of the abilities that doctors need for all domains of medical practice (Frank, Snell & Sherbino, 2015). The framework illustrates that the doctor role is not a single role but a multiplicity of roles. Roles are communicator, collaborator, leader, health advocate, scholar, professional, and the integrating role of medical expert, as shown in Figure 6. Associated with each of these roles are competencies linked to essential tasks of practice. For example, within the medical expert role, essential tasks include history taking, examination, diagnosis and management, and within the communication role, essential tasks are conducting a patient-centred interview and documenting clinical encounters.

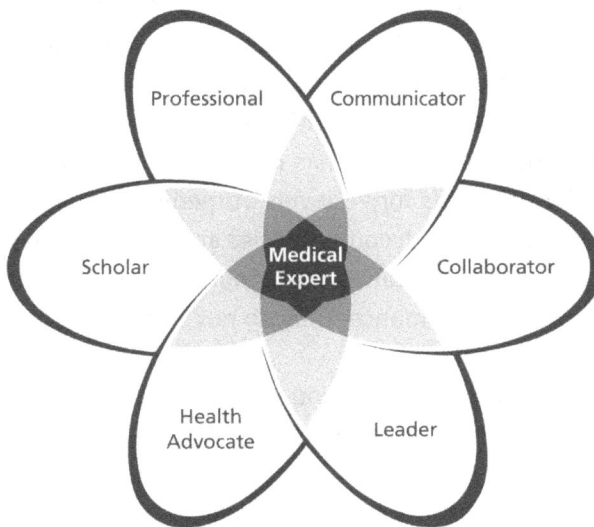

Figure 6. The CanMEDS Framework
Source: Frank, J.R., Snell, L., & Sherbino, J. (Eds.) (2015).
Copyright © 2015 The Royal College of Physicians and Surgeons of Canada. Reproduced with permission.

Performance of essential tasks to the required level

Meeting performance indicators

For the doctor in practice, the expected or required level of performance of essential tasks is associated with the doctor's seniority or stage of training. A minimum level of performance can be specified but a maximum level cannot, as performance of essential tasks in representative task conditions occurs on a continuum and performance can potentially continue to improve. Common indicators of performance, such as peer or patient feedback and chart audits may be used as performance benchmarks and rough measures of relative expertise. Training programs usually have their own standards for performance. However, some performance may not fit with established indicators, particularly if the performance pertains to innovative and creative advances, and involves new techniques that redefine performance (Weisberg, 2006). Patient safety is paramount: "a fundamental minimum requirement of all clinicians is that they be safe practitioners" (Ahern, Morley & McColl, 2016, p. 374).

Deploying competencies

Another way of thinking about performing essential tasks to the required level is deployment of competencies. Competencies are observable, measurable and assessable abilities or characteristics that are required for practice. They can be reliably and reproducibly assessed against a commonly agreed standard (AMA, 2010). For this reason, the assessment of competencies has become commonplace in both medical training programs and in hospitals for all levels of medical, nursing and allied health staff. Training can equip a doctor with competencies and the necessary conditioning for deploying competencies in representative task conditions. While competencies are an important starting point for performance, they do not ensure performance.

> "The distinction between competence and performance is important.
> Competence can be defined as 'what the doctor has been trained to do.'
> It involves acquiring and maintaining the requisite knowledge, skills and
> behaviours to perform at or above minimum standard. Performance can be
> defined as 'what the doctor actually does from day to day'."
> (Royal Australasian College of Physicians, 2010, p.6)

A doctor may possess demonstrated knowledge and skills and be certified as competent in controlled assessment scenarios, but if they fail to apply their knowledge and skills to clinical scenarios and the reality of the patients before them, they fail to perform. Competencies must be integrated into the comprehensive care of a wide range of patients and in various settings (AMA, 2010).

Adapting in response to demands

The integration of competencies in the care of patients involves adaptations. Feltovich, Prietula and Ericsson (2006) explain the link between expertise and adaptations as follows.

> "Expertise is appropriately viewed not as simple (and often short-term) matter of fact or skill acquisition, but rather as a complex construct of adaptations of mind and body which include substantial self-monitoring and control mechanisms, to task environments in service of representative task goals and activities." (p.57)

The doctor is required to adapt to an infinite variety of patient needs, and task goals and conditions. This is true of procedures (e.g. when there is anatomical or physiological variations) and of non-procedural medicine (e.g. tailoring complex cancer treatment to patients from rural areas who may be unable to travel).

Only the most straightforward tasks are carried out according to simple rules or through automaticity. Experts start with a performance goal, execute and monitor the performance in order to detect problems, and evaluate and select alternative actions continuously during performance in order to track and pursue achievement of the performance goal (Ericsson, 2015).

Performance in a manner appropriate to the setting

Understanding and solving health problems within a setting

With patients and team members, the doctor has to co-construct what constitutes a problem to be solved, and formulate the response to problems as defined tasks and plans. Performance has to occur within a defined or reasonable period of time to be acceptable for all involved, for example, the doctor, the patient, the patients who are waiting, and the nursing staff. Though often unavoidable, delays in certain areas of practice (e.g. a theatre list) may result in numerous consequences and costs, such as patient distress, staff overtime and excess cost to the healthcare system. As such, time is often used as a measure of performance, and "expertise transcends how individual tasks are accomplished, to involve how time is made accountably productive" (Clancey, 2006, p. 137).

An example of the need to define what constitutes a problem to be solved and to make time accountably productive in a manner appropriate to the setting is the emergency department. With high-throughput, high-acuity care, emergency departments are often necessarily cursory when it comes to chronic health issues. A conscientious intern may wish to address the patient's cholesterol after they have come in for a broken foot, but this would not constitute appropriate performance in the setting – speed is a priority, and dealing with non-urgent chronic health issues should be left in the hands of the general practitioner.

Noticing and responding appropriately to the socio-spatial dimensions of work

The socio-spatial dimensions of work are the interactions between people, and people and their surroundings at work. Clancy's (2006) metaphor of a stage show, with many participants involved in contributing to the quality of the performance, reveals the socio-spatial dimensions of the work of a doctor. The doctor has work to perform (roles to play), and surrounding the doctor is the stage (the setting), acts (blocks of work or shifts), seasons of performance (performance in response to health conditions occurring in seasonal patterns), an audience (patients and bystanders), and other cast (peers within the community of practice). Not everything happens on stage, considering how the doctor prepares, who assists, how they get information regarding the day's work, where and when they review and plan work in off-stage areas, and how events are scheduled. The socio-spatial dimensions have implications for the work of a doctor. Many variables, such as ward processes, generate specific performance requirements, and many variables, such as the multidisciplinary team, provide resources.

Beyond the immediate surroundings of the doctor are a multitude of contextual influences on practice. To notice the influences and how they interact, consider the work of the doctor in nested contexts beyond the room, within a clinic, within a hospital, within a health service, within a state, and beyond. Figure 7 illustrates some of the many interacting influences on practice including rostering, the multidisciplinary team, workplace culture, technology, regulatory agencies and corporate entities.

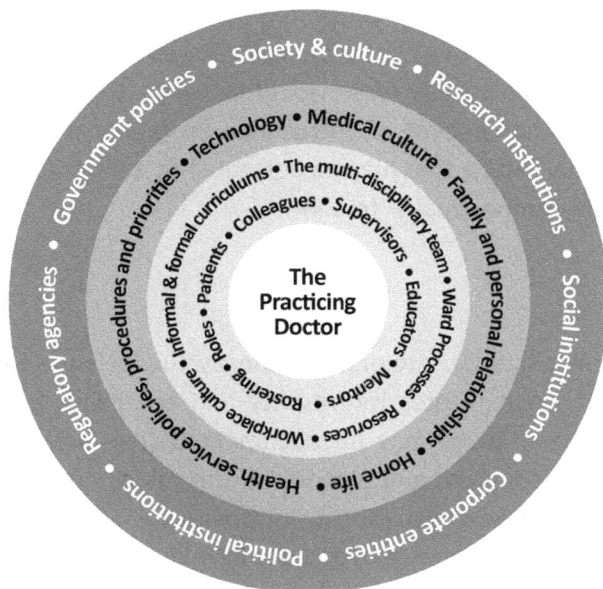

Figure 7. Interacting influences on practice

Performance in accordance with regulations

Abiding by codes of conduct, laws and by-laws

Various legislative, regulatory and organisational requirements apply to the work of the doctor. Codes of conduct such as the Good Medical Practice: A Code of Conduct for Doctors in Australia (Medical Board of Australia, 2014) describe what constitutes proper, professional and ethical conduct, and what is expected of practicing doctors by peers and the patient community. Codes of conduct may be written into laws of states and countries, and by-laws of health services. An array of policies, procedures and protocols also apply within health services.

Working within a scope of practice

Scope of practice refers to the boundaries of the doctor's practice, containing acceptable and permitted tasks and processes. Usually scope of practice is derived from competency-based assessment that measures what the doctor can demonstrably do in controlled representations of professional practice, or from assessment of performance in practice. Scope of practice may have conditions attached, such as the need to practice with a specific level of supervision for particular tasks. An area related to scope of practice is *Entrustable Professional Activities*. CanMEDS (Frank, Snell and Sherbino, 2015) uses the concept of Entrustable Professional Activities to describe "tasks in a professional setting that may be delegated to a physician once competency in that task has been demonstrated" (p. 28).

Enacting values

Many health agencies promote core organisational values to unite workers in a shared commitment to values (e.g. integrity, respect and reliability) and the behaviours reflecting those values. Values may be documented (e.g. within job descriptions, values statements and charters) and embodying the values may be a requirement of employment. When the doctor consciously internalises and embodies the values, the values contribute to self-regulation and guide principled action on a consistent basis.

An example of a charter is the Charter of Medical Professionalism (ABIM Foundation, ACP-ASIM Foundation, & European Federation of Internal Medicine, 2002). The charter promotes three principles of professionalism; primacy of patient welfare (serving interests of patients), patient autonomy (empowering patients to make informed decisions), and social justice (eliminating discrimination, and fair distribution of resources), and ten associated commitments.

Knowing, doing and being in the medical profession

Another way to view the work of a doctor in practice is in terms of knowing, doing and being, introduced in Chapter 1, p.5. These dimensions are similar to 'knows', 'knows how', 'shows how', 'does' and 'is' proposed by Cruess, Cruess and Steinert (2016) in their adaptation of Miller's Pyramid (Miller, 1990). Knowing relates to possessing a dynamic knowledge base of relevant facts, concepts and skills for doing the work of a doctor in a particular setting and context. Doing relates to applying the acquired knowledge and skills in an intelligent way to meet the healthcare needs of patients served. Being relates to consciously enacting a values base for practice that integrates personal values and the values of the medical profession. All three dimensions are essential for scientific, humanistic medical practice.

In an integrated and fluid repertoire of knowing, doing and being, knowing informs being and doing, being drives knowing and doing, and doing consolidates and challenges knowing and being, as shown in Figure 8. In a disintegrated repertoire there are gaps between knowing, doing and being. A gap between knowing and doing means that knowledge is not applied. A gap between being and doing means behaviours may be at odds with personal and professional values and may lack foundation in ethical practice. A gap between being and knowing means valuable knowledge is not pursued.

The essential task of hand washing illustrates these ideas. A doctor working with infectious patients has detailed handwashing protocol knowledge and skills (knowing), follows the protocols (doing), and upholds their commitment to being a safe doctor (being). Disintegration in their repertoire of knowing, doing and being in relation to handwashing (e.g. the doctor knowing but not applying handwashing protocols), causes a disintegration in the safety and quality of healthcare.

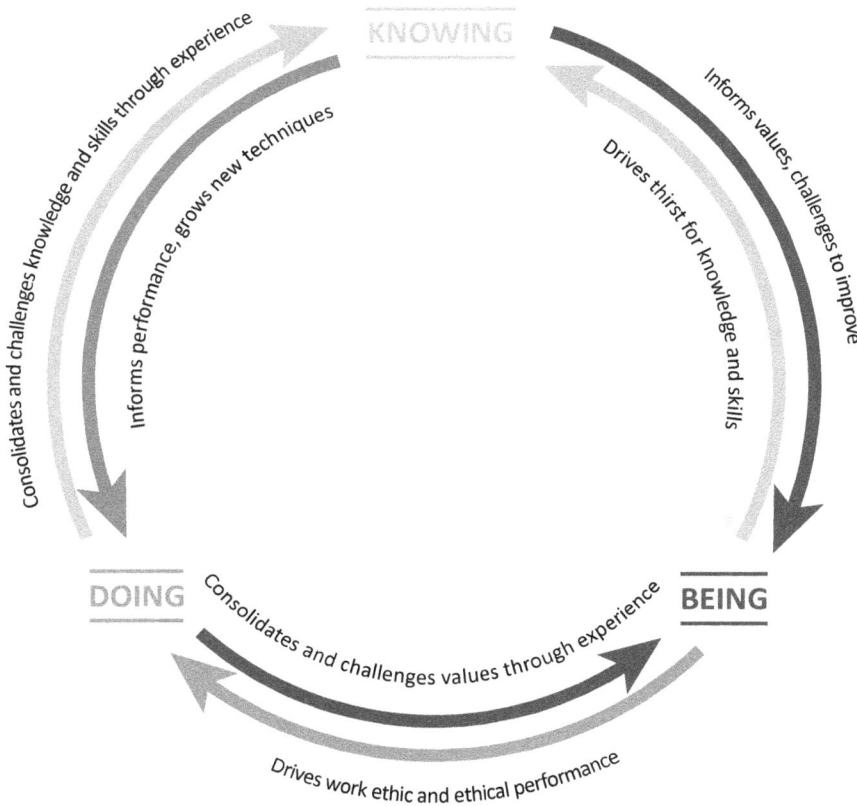

Figure 8. Three dimensions of scientific, humanistic medical practice

Developing as a doctor

The three dimensions of knowing, doing and being are also useful for illuminating aspects of developing as a doctor in practice. Developing as a doctor in practice and functioning optimally in a particular context encompasses development of all three dimensions. The three dimensions are relevant to all doctors in practice, irrespective of seniority, job description, specialty, context and setting. During clinical training years, acquiring knowledge, skills, performance, and awareness and practise of values occurs gradually over time (for a theoretical account of skill development and the doctor's developmental journey, *see* Appendix A, pp.191–5 and Appendix B, pp.197–9). After clinical training, acquired knowledge, skills and performance must be actively maintained to prevent decline. Furthermore, the nature of health organisations as complex adaptive systems means that all areas of practice, including patient expectations, medical technology, health service policies and procedures, and best practice, are subject to change, requiring participants within the system to continue developing and adapting.

From the perspective of the mentor, attention to the three dimensions of development adds focus to developmental work with the mentee. In Chapter 4, p.42–8 targets of developmental work are derived from the three dimensions of development and the four themes in the work of a doctor in practice.

3. Developmental needs of doctors

What are doctors' developmental needs?

The doctor development strategies described in Chapter 1, pp.6–8 are channels for resources that benefit the doctor in their pursuit of development. We refer to resources external to the doctor that benefit their development as *developmental needs*, and classify the needs as support, challenge and facilitation by the effect that they have on the doctor. A key part of the mentor's role is to recognise and address the mentee's developmental needs for support, challenge and facilitation, as the mentee sets and achieves goals, navigates their clinical training system, adapts to the demands of their job, and encounter the uncertainties of medical practice.

As a prelude to coverage of the mentor's role in Chapter 4, p.41 and the mentor's toolkit in Part 2, the focus of this chapter is on recognising the developmental needs of the doctor who is a mentee. A chapter is devoted to this topic, because the mentor's ability to recognise developmental needs of the mentee is a prerequisite to addressing developmental needs.

Support

Support in relation to developmental needs of mentees refers to strengthening resources benefiting the mentee in their development. Being a doctor and developing as a doctor in practice takes strength, particularly at times of encountering uncertainty, adapting to unfamiliar environments, facing indecision and fear, resolving conflict, and managing grief and loss. Qualities that are strengthened with support include self-belief, calmness, clarity, a sense of direction, motivation, stamina and will. Offering support encompasses many types of assistance, for example, exploring the mentee's ideas about the doctor they want to become, reassuring and validating, sharing experiences and resources, and responding to vulnerability with kindness.

Challenge

Challenge in relation to developmental needs of mentees refers to strain-inducing resources benefiting the mentee in their development. When delivered constructively, challenge provides the mentee with stimulation to develop, particularly in relation to skilled performance of essential tasks of practice. By rising to challenge, doctors go beyond their comfort zone, and acquire cognitive and physiological mechanisms for producing and controlling performance, and improving performance (*see* Appendix A, pp.191–5). Examples of providing challenge are asking difficult questions, describing the next level of difficulty of an essential task, giving feedback on performance, suggesting techniques and methods for improving performance, and following up on the mentee's fulfilment of commitments. In many areas of medical practice, challenges do not need to be created, as they are an existing reality of practice in a complex adaptive system. Existing challenges are useful catalysts of development.

Facilitation

Facilitation in relation to developmental needs of mentees refers to breakthrough-enabling resources benefiting the mentee in their development. Facilitation provides momentum at times when the mentee has become stuck and or when accelerated progress by the mentee is desired. Facilitation may have a range of intended outcomes, for example, learning of knowledge and skills, gaining insight, problem solving and decision making. Types of assistance that involve facilitation include teaching, debriefing, sharing experiences and resources, introducing the mentee to colleagues, and assisting the mentee to translate their ideas into actionable goals and steps towards goal achievement.

Table 3 describes common developmental needs of mentees for support, challenge and facilitation.

Table 3. Common developmental needs of mentees for support, challenge and facilitation

CATEGORY OF DEVELOPMENTAL NEED	COMMON DEVELOPMENTAL NEEDS
Support strengthening resources	Feedback that is 'off the radar' and outside formal assessment processes Reassurance and validation Honest and open discussion about the mentee including their strengths and vulnerabilities A space for exploring options and making decisions A space for honest examination of practices and testing knowledge safely A space for the mentee to find an answer to the question – 'Am I doing okay?' An ally who believes in them Guidance on how to be a doctor in a specific setting or context Recognition of achievements Encouragement
Challenge strain-inducing resources	Information about the next level of performance to strive for Opportunities to practice at the next level of performance under appropriate supervision Experiences relevant to current and future roles Questions to the mentee, about their values, choices and priorities Accountability conversations about following through on decisions and commitments Review of performance and feedback Access to activities allowing repetition, error detection and correction Invitations to confront avoidance and make decisions Invitations to apply knowledge and skills to challenging clinical scenarios
Facilitation breakthrough-enabling resources	Access to activities likely to be important in acquiring new knowledge and skills Assistance with overcoming obstacles Assistance with finding connections between past experiences and new challenges Assistance with discovering the applications of knowledge and skills Assistance with recognising work to be done Referrals to other helpers Dialogue about local culture and policies applicable to the mentee's work Conversations for making sense of difficult situations Conversations for learning knowledge and skills Conversations for increasing insight Conversations for building and sustaining resilience

Sources of information about the mentee's needs for support, challenge and facilitation

Bradshaw's taxonomy of social need (Bradshaw, 1972) describes need in four categories by how the need is revealed. Applied to mentoring, the taxonomy guides the mentor's recognition of developmental needs of mentees, such as those displayed in Table 3. The four sources of information about developmental needs of mentees are:

1. *Felt need*, what the mentee says they need. This is determined by the mentee, and may be related to either mandatory or chosen aspects of the aspirational state of development. Examples of felt need are: the mentee stating that they need an opportunity to participate in a clinical task at a higher level of difficulty (challenge); access to the multidisciplinary team (support); and guidance on synthesising assessment information into a differential diagnosis (facilitation of clinical reasoning skill development).
2. *Normative need*, what a credible authority says the mentee needs. This type of need often relates to mandatory aspects of an aspirational state of development. Examples of normative need are CanMEDS describing milestones applicable to each level of seniority (challenge), *beyondblue* recommending that all doctors have a general practitioner (support), and the Australian Medical Council requiring all interns to receive feedback on performance (facilitation of insight).
3. *Comparative need*, a need revealed through the services required by a similar population of doctors. Examples of comparative need are: a doctor in an Emergency Department needing similar access to critical incident debriefing (support) as a doctor within another Emergency Department; a surgical registrar needing to be supervised performing the same number of procedures as their peers before being allowed to perform a procedure solo (challenge); and a doctor rostered to work in one rural facility needing the same training (facilitation of learning) as a doctor rostered to work in a similar rural facility.
4. *Expressed need*, a need demonstrated through the uptake of services. Examples of expressed need are: the need for confidential debriefing (support) demonstrated through uptake of counselling services; the need for simulation training (challenge) demonstrated through participation in simulation events; and the need for training in interview preparation (facilitation of learning) demonstrated through the number of doctors applying for interview skills courses.

The four sources of information about developmental needs of mentees are illustrated in Figure 9.

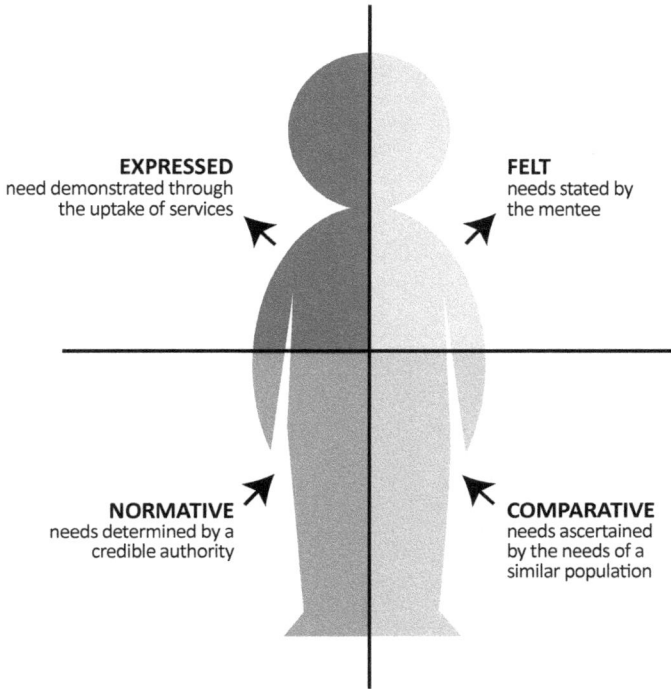

EXPRESSED
need demonstrated through
the uptake of services

FELT
needs stated by
the mentee

NORMATIVE
needs determined by a
credible authority

COMPARATIVE
needs ascertained
by the needs of a
similar population

Figure 9. Four sources of information about the mentee's developmental needs

Tailoring support, challenge and facilitation to the individual mentee

Every mentee is an individual, with their own history, circumstances, aspirational state of development, goals, and needs for various types of support, challenge and facilitation. A major advantage of intentional mentoring as a strategy for doctor development is that it provides the mentee with personalised assistance as they pursue developmental outcomes that are meaningful to them. In intentional mentoring, there is good fit between the support, challenge and facilitation that the mentee needs, and the support, challenge and facilitation that the mentor provides. In Chapter 4, pp.48–9 and Chapter 5, pp.63-4 the focus turns to the mentor's perspective of support, challenge and facilitation, as types of influence exerted by the mentor to foster development.

4. The intentional mentor's role

Facets of the role

Previous chapters have viewed mentoring from the perspective of both the mentor and the mentee: intentional mentoring is a purpose-driven partnership and process (or strategy) for development, and both the mentor and the mentee contribute through relational and developmental work. This chapter focuses on the mentor's portion of the relational and developmental work, and describes the mentor role in terms of its three main facets:

- Doing relational work
- Doing developmental work
- Giving structure to mentoring

The guiding principles of intentional mentoring, constructiveness (relating positively) and productivity (doing more of what works for the mentee's development), apply to the mentor's role. The intentional mentor aims to foster development through relating positively and delivering individually-relevant support, challenge and facilitation as described in Chapter 3, p.35.

Doing relational work

The first facet of the mentor role is doing relational work, work to build relationship. The relational work of the mentor covers four main areas, commitment (being committed), accessibility (being accessible), responsiveness (being responsive) and engagement (being engaged). A memory aid for the relational work of the mentor, is CARE, an extension of the work of Johnson (2008) who described the importance of accessibility, responsiveness and engagement (ARE) in creating strong bonds between partners.

Commitment – By accepting the role of mentor you are making a commitment to be a resource to the mentee for a time and a purpose related to the mentee's development. The specific details of the commitment depend on the agreement you form with the mentee and typically include a commitment to providing a level of accessibility, responsiveness and engagement.

Accessibility – Being accessible to the mentee means being available to them, being open to them contacting you, and being reasonably easy to reach at agreed times.

Responsiveness – Being responsive to the mentee includes replying to the mentee's questions, giving feedback in response to their actions, and responding to contact (e.g. text messages and emails) in a timely way.

Engagement – Engaging with the mentee refers to having a connection with the mentee. The ultimate form of connection is empathy, having a sense of what the mentee is experiencing, what matters most to them, and their perspective of issues. With engagement, you avoid generic and irrelevant responses to the mentee. Authentic engagement is a two-way connection and is enhanced when the mentor and mentee choose to be genuine and honest with one another about strengths and vulnerabilities.

In mentoring, CARE increases the likelihood of a bond conducive to a sound mentoring partnership and process, and the achievement of desired outcomes. A summary of the relational work of the mentor is included in Table 4.

Table 4. The relational work of the mentor

RELATIONAL WORK	
Mentee's work Trust the mentor Honour commitments	**Mentor's work** Be trustworthy CARE, be committed, accessible, responsive and engaged
Work shared by the mentor and the mentee Accept responsibilities, fulfil commitments and adjust the partnership as the mentee develops or as circumstances change	

Doing developmental work

The second facet of the mentor role is doing developmental work, work to foster development. The *scope* or range of developmental work is work that contributes to the mentee's development as a doctor in practice. The *focus* of the work is assisting the mentee to set and achieve meaningful goals.

The scope of developmental work: contributing to the mentee's development as a doctor in practice

Assisting the mentee to acquire knowledge and skills, performance, and awareness and practise of values

The scope of developmental work is generally broad; it includes assisting the mentee to acquire knowledge and skills, performance, and awareness and practise of values, relevant to their job, career path and aspirations in the medical profession. During negotiation of the mentoring partnership, mentors may wish to delineate a narrower scope of developmental work.

Table 5 displays possible targets of developmental work, based on the four themes in the work of a doctor in practice described in Chapter 2, pp.26–7:

- performance of roles for meeting the healthcare needs of patients served,
- to the required level of performance of essential tasks,
- in a manner appropriate to the setting, and
- in accordance with regulations.

Methods for assisting the mentee to acquire knowledge and skills, performance, and awareness and practise of values, are covered in Part Two (*see* Chapter 7, pp.81–91, Chapter 8, pp.93–5, Chapter 9, pp.97–100, and Chapter 10, pp.101–110) and the Appendices section (*see* Appendix H, pp.219–224 and Appendix I, pp.225–7).

Table 5. Fostering doctor development

DIMENSION OF DEVELOPMENT	TARGETS OF DEVELOPMENTAL WORK
Knowing Acquiring knowledge and skills	***Roles*** Developing knowledge, skills and competencies required for the performance of essential tasks and roles
	Level of performance Understanding the expected level of performance
	Increasing the knowledge and skills base and competencies required for higher level performance
	Preparing for entry to the next stage of training
	Practice setting Understanding setting-specific parameters of practice
	Developing role clarity
	Preparing for uncommon presentations and non-routine performance conditions
	Regulations Understanding legislative, regulatory and organisational requirements

Doing Acquiring performance	*Roles* Acquiring and improving or maintaining performance of essential tasks within the roles of communicator, collaborator, leader, health advocate, scholar, professional and medical expert (the CanMEDS roles)
	Level of performance Meeting performance indicators and achieving targets
	Practice settings Adapting and responding effectively to setting-specific challenges
	Translating competency in controlled settings to proficiency in practice settings
	Regulations and standards Following laws, policies, procedures, protocols and guidelines
Being Acquiring awareness and practise of values, across all areas of practice	Embodying roles (e.g. the CanMEDS roles) and chosen qualities of practice including resilience
	Forming a concept of self as a doctor
	Combining aspects of one's professional self, e.g. knowledge and skills, with aspects of one's personal self, e.g. cultural background and life experiences
	Integrating and enacting personal values and values of the profession
	Forming commitments
	Identifying, reconciling and prioritising values in daily practice
	Anticipating and being prepared for value conflicts and for moral and ethical dilemmas under pressure
	Finding purpose in being a doctor

Assisting the mentee to acquire relevant knowledge and skills, performance, and awareness and practise of values, may involve other endeavours including the following.

Making every day work practices visible

The mentee's work performance relies on recognising work to be done. "When everyone in a community shares a habit, it ordinarily becomes invisible, for what everyone does no one easily recognises" (Engeström, 1999, p. 63). For a mentee arriving in a work area, many aspects of the work are not immediately visible to them. *Visibilization* of work is the term Engeström uses for attempts to make everyday practices of work visible. A mentor with experience of a work area can make everyday practices of work visible and reveal the socio-spatial dimensions of the work that are invisible to newcomers, yet significant to practice.

Making influences on work performance visible

For the practicing doctor, performance involves recognising and overcoming barriers to practice, and the mentor can assist. Miller's Pyramid, a popular framework for assessment of clinical skills, competence and performance (Miller, 1990), contains an implicit assumption that competence predicts performance. The Cambridge Model (Rethans et al., 2002), an adaptation of Miller's Pyramid, illustrates that performance is actually a product of competence combined with system and individual influences on performance, as shown in Figure 10. A mentor can assist to illuminate the many system and individual influences on the mentee's practice, including barriers and enablers of performance.

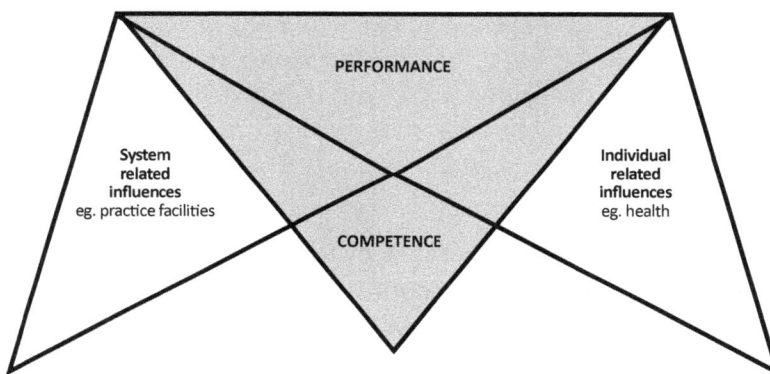

Figure 10. The Cambridge Model
Source: Rethans, et al. (2002)

Encouraging job knowledge and tacit knowledge gains

Job knowledge is the vast knowledge base explicitly taught in preparation for practice. Tacit knowledge is knowledge learned on the job via experience, and is not explicitly taught. It involves understanding the 'what' and the 'why' of action at a particular time (Cianciolo, Matthew, Sternberg & Wagner, 2006). In medical practice, a list of differential diagnoses for chest pain is an example of job knowledge; applying this knowledge in the care of a patient presenting with chest pain and arriving at an appropriate diagnosis and treatment is tacit knowledge. Together, job and tacit knowledge are used by doctors in the performance of their work and "the interplay between formal knowledge of medicine and experiential knowledge has emerged as a central issue in understanding medical expertise" (Norman, Eva, Brooks & Hamstra, 2006, p.340). The mentor assists the mentee to access opportunities that allow growth in both job knowledge and experiential knowledge.

Providing practice opportunities for situated learning

A source of experiential knowledge is situated learning. While classroom learning involves acquiring knowledge out of context and frequently in an abstract form, situated learning involves learning within the work context and during the performance of work. The premise of situated learning is that learning and doing co-occur within *communities of practice*, defined as "groups of people who share a concern or a passion for something they do and learn how to do it better as they interact regularly" (Wenger-Trayner & Wenger-Trayner, 2015, p.1). A new member of a community of practice enters the community with a certain level of knowledge and skills and begins to have peripheral participation. As they learn the behaviours, values and norms of the community of practice and become increasingly active and engaged, they take on more central roles (Lave & Wenger, 1991). The mentor assists the mentee to form helpful connections and progressively take on more central roles in the community of practice.

Guiding reflective enquiry

"The practice of medicine is distinguished by the need for judgement in the face of uncertainty. Doctors take responsibility for these judgements and their consequences. A doctor's up-to-date knowledge and skill provide the explicit scientific and often tacit experiential basis for such judgements. But because so much of medicine's unpredictability calls for wisdom as well as technical ability, doctors are vulnerable to the charge that their decisions are neither transparent nor accountable. In an age where deference is dead and league tables are the norm, doctors must be clearer about what they do, and how and why they do it."
(Royal College of Physicians of London, 2005, p.xi)

Reflective enquiry enables the mentee to be clearer about what they do, and how and why they do it. The essence of reflective enquiry is directing attention and awareness to one's own thinking, actions and experiences, to acquire:

- knowledge – consolidation of knowledge, creation of knowledge (including deep learning from experience) and retention of knowledge
- insight – noticing internal processes, being aware of assumptions and motivations underlying practice, finding relationships between what took place and what resulted, and identifying multiple perspectives of a situation or problem

- resolutions, decisions and commitments – resolving discordance between personal values and cultural norms, deciding what and how to change in the future to improve practice, and adopting thoughtful, carefully considered practices as an alternative to automatic or impulsive practices.

The mentor assists the mentee to acquire knowledge, insight, resolutions, decisions and commitments through guiding reflective enquiry. For examples of reflective enquiry prompts, as well as a guide to fostering metacognition (thinking about thinking), *see* Appendix C, pp.201–4.

Assisting at points of transition

Key points of transition in a doctor's developmental journey from intern to consultant (e.g. from medical student to intern, or registrar to consultant), require extensive adaptation. During times of transition the mentor helps the mentee to:

- find their feet – gain a sense of being grounded, steady and prepared, by understanding the work to be done and the resources available, both internal resources (e.g. knowledge and skills) and external resources (e.g. multidisciplinary team members and equipment)
- find their way – sort through competing priorities and gain a sense of direction for what matters most (e.g. priorities for service delivery and learning and growth)
- find themselves as a doctor – gain clarity about their role and professional identity or self-concept as a doctor (e.g. integrating what they know, what they do, what their values are, and the roles they play, into a concept of self as a doctor).

Advocating

The developmental work of the mentor may include advocacy. The mentor may advocate for the mentee's access to improved work conditions, resources and developmental opportunities. They may also facilitate the mentee's own efforts to advocate for what they or others need, and to initiate change within the complex adaptive system of healthcare.

The focus of developmental work: assisting the mentee to set and achieve goals aligned with their aspirational state of development

The developmental work focuses on identifying the mentee's aspirational state of development, setting aligned goals for development (an initial goal may be to identify or formulate an aspirational state of development to set parameters for goal setting), and understanding and responding to the mentee's needs for support, challenge and facilitation as they pursue goal achievement. This work assists the mentee to achieve their goals and advance towards their aspirational state of development.

A summary of the developmental work of the mentor is included in Table 6.

Table 6. The developmental work of the mentor

DEVELOPMENTAL WORK	
Mentee's work	**Mentor's work**
Describe their aspirational state of development	Help the mentee to figure out their aspirational state of development
Choose goals to pursue in mentoring, aligned with their aspirational state of development	Assist the mentee to translate their aspirational state of development to goals
Describe what they need from the mentor	Recognise and respond to the developmental needs of the mentee for support, challenge and facilitation, in service of their goals
Work shared by the mentor and the mentee	
Understand mentoring goals and have goal-directed interactions	

Giving structure to mentoring

The third facet of the mentor role is giving structure to mentoring. Structure is required to carry out the principles and practices of intentional mentoring, and to ensure that the purpose and anticipated course of mentoring is clear. The mentor gives structure to both the mentoring partnership and process for development. In structuring the partnership, the mentor oversees the formation of the partnership, the collaboration and the parting of ways at the conclusion of mentoring. In structuring the process for development, the mentor oversees the translation of the mentee's aspirational state of development into goals, and goals into goal-directed interactions.

While giving structure to mentoring, the mentor considers balance, for example, balance in the amount of challenge, support and facilitation they provide. Too much support without enough challenge could limit the development of the mentee. Too much challenge without support could result in partnership breakdown. Too much facilitation without enough challenge could create dependency. Another type of balance to consider is the amount of attention to the mentee's past, present and future. Attention to each time zone offers keys to development: the past holds lessons for the future, the present holds choices and opportunities to live meaningfully now, and the future holds possibilities for what might be. A third example is balance in the amount of attention to acquisition of knowing, doing and being, and integration of these dimensions. This balance is necessary for holistic development that leads to scientific and humanistic medical practice.

The mentor role is not the doctor role

The doctor role is a multiplicity of roles, as is the mentor role. Aspects of the mentor role include coach, confidante, counsellor and educator. The role of doctor providing medical care is not part of the mentor role. While mentoring practice and medical practice share some common ground, such as identifying and responding to needs, the two areas of practice have significant differences. One of the differences is how expertise is regarded. In medical practice, the doctor is typically regarded as the expert in the partnership. In mentoring practice, the mentee is regarded as an expert who can find solutions and a way forward with the support of the mentor (Doherty, 2004). While the mentor may have more expertise in the domain of medicine, the mentee has more expertise in the domain of their life, and in recognising what types of assistance are most helpful to them.

Who can be a mentor?

According to our definition of mentoring, mentoring occurs in a voluntary partnership between two professionals with a difference in experience of professional practice. Therefore, all doctors can potentially become mentors to doctors who have less experience. Mentor and mentee duos may include:

- an intern and a medical student
- an intern and another intern with more experience of healthcare, such as a previous background in pharmacy or nursing
- a resident and an intern
- a senior resident/registrar and a resident

- a consultant and registrar
- a consultant and a junior consultant
- a retired consultant and retiring consultant.

The difference in experience between the mentor and the mentee becomes less pronounced as the mentee grows in experience. The mentee may eventually outgrow the partnership. This is a normal and natural part of mentoring.

Having identical career paths is not a necessity for the mentor and mentee. For example, a gastroenterologist can mentor a cardiology resident. Clinical process, more so than knowledge, is transmitted during mentoring. The mentor role allows for referrals to others for different aspects of the developmental work when required.

Mentor attributes

To be able to perform the three facets of the mentor role effectively, helpful attributes are as follows.

Willingness and goodwill

The relational and developmental work of mentoring requires your willingness and deliberate investment of goodwill. Willingness and goodwill are demonstrated through CARE, behaviours reflecting commitment, accessibility, responsiveness and engagement. The antithesis of CARE is MEAN, behaviours reflecting malice, ego, agenda and negativity, each hazardous for the relational and developmental work of mentoring.

Positive role modeling

As a mentor and a senior doctor, even when you are not actively involved in goal-directed interaction, you are a role model. You have a continuous influence on colleagues either positively or negatively through your example and modeling of behaviours. You are likely to have an influence on many colleagues at a low level of influence, an influence on some colleagues at a moderate level of influence, and an influence on a few colleagues at a high level of influence, for example, in your work with mentees. Aim to have a positive influence, wherever possible.

Genuineness

One of the characteristics of an effective helper is being genuine (Egan, 2002), particularly in your interest in the mentee and their development. Genuine interest can encourage the mentee to engage more often in mentoring activities and to pursue developmental outcomes with confidence that someone believes in them and their abilities. Being genuine is also about being authentic in the partnership, honest about your strengths and vulnerabilities, and aware of what you are bringing to the partnership. You are more relatable if you are willing to reveal your real self.

Performance and participation

Having sound performance as a doctor, and continuing involvement in activities for your own development as a doctor, gives you credibility as a mentor, and resources to draw on for mentoring. You may choose to engage in mentoring as a mentee as well as a mentor. Having experience as a mentee offers you an additional avenue of development as a mentor, through your mentor's role modeling.

Possessing knowledge, skills and tools for the mentor role

Knowledge, skills and tools are required as a foundation for mentoring practice. For a sample mentor role description summarising the knowledge, skills and tools promoted in this book, *see* Appendix D, pp.205–7.

An approach to performing the role of intentional mentor: I-Mentor with the Cycle of Caring

In Chapter 1, pp.12–13 we introduced the Model of Intentional Mentoring as a representation of intentional mentoring practices, that is, the relational and developmental work of the mentor and the mentee. By incorporating a classic model of helping partnerships, the Cycle of Caring (Skovholt, 2005) with the Model of Intentional Mentoring, we represent the mentor's portion of the relational and development work of intentional mentoring in an approach we call I-Mentor with the Cycle of Caring.

I-Mentor with the Cycle of Caring: stages of mentoring

Skovholt proposes that an effective helping partnership will progress through three key stages, collectively known as the Cycle of Caring. The stages, applied to mentoring, are as follows.

- *Empathic attachment* – The essence of empathic attachment is an open-minded attitude by the mentor; a trusting, collaborative alliance with the right balance between professional under-attachment and over-attachment.
- *Active involvement* – The essence of active involvement is consistent, sustained caring for the mentee; sharing a vision of development and progress and working towards it.
- *Felt separation* – The essence of felt separation is a letting go of active emotional commitments; separating well and being energised in preparation for future mentoring partnerships.

Illustrated in Figure 11, the combination of the Model of Intentional Mentoring and the Cycle of Caring to form I-Mentor with the Cycle of Caring offers clarity on where to place your focus throughout mentoring; empathic attachment, active involvement and felt separation become landmarks for your mentoring practice.

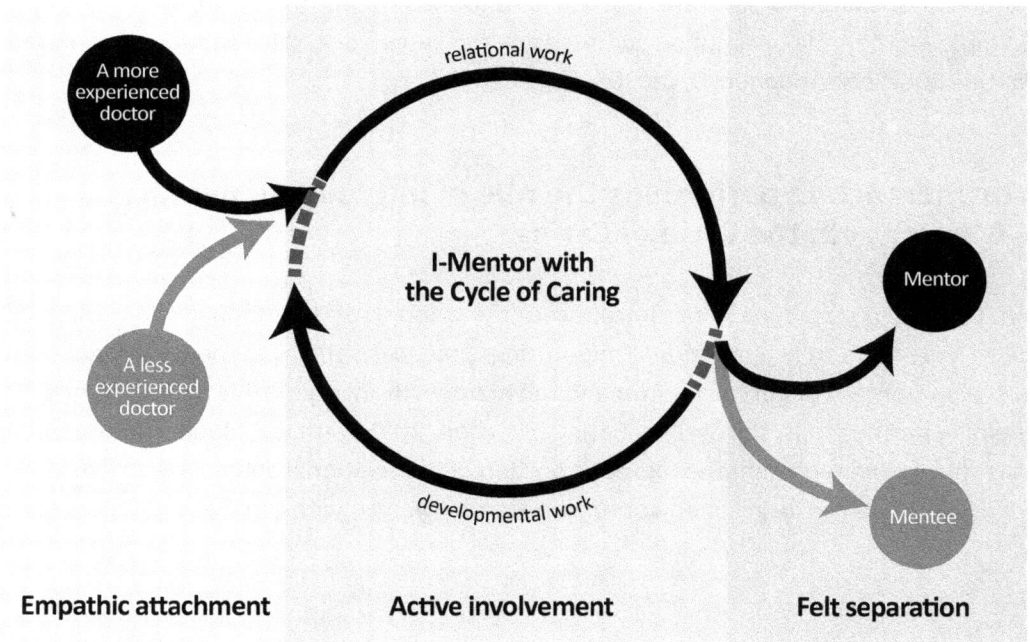

Figure 11. I-Mentor with the Cycle of Caring

During the empathic attachment stage, you form a trusting partnership with the mentee. During the active involvement stage, you collaborate on the mentee's development, and adjust the partnership and responsibilities as the mentee develops and or circumstances change. During the felt separation stage, you part ways positively. Your mentoring tasks at each stage are described in Table 7.

Table 7. Mentoring tasks by stage

STAGE	MENTORING TASKS
Empathic attachment Essence: an open-minded attitude by the mentor; a trusting, collaborative alliance with the right balance between professional under-attachment and over-attachment.	Build trust Identify mentoring goal/s aligning with the mentee's aspirational state of development Agree to work together as mentor and mentee
Active involvement Essence: consistent, sustained caring for the mentee; sharing a vision of development and progress and working towards it.	Identify an agenda for each session Work collaboratively on goal achievement Notice results Do more of what works for the mentee's development and movement towards their aspirational state of development Re-negotiate the partnership as the mentee develops or as circumstances change
Felt separation Essence: letting go of active emotional commitments; separating well and being energised in preparation for future mentoring partnerships.	Recognise achievements Decide to conclude mentoring End the partnership on a positive note

I-Mentor with the Cycle of Caring: the intentional mentor's toolkit

A *tool* is something that helps to perform a job or get work done. The work done by the intentional mentor is relational work and developmental work, and ten tools are key to this work. The tools are purposeful communication, partnership, goal-directed interaction, curriculum and performance standards, brief intervention, resilience work, career guidance, confidentiality, evaluation and reflective practice of mentoring. Collectively, they are called the intentional mentor's toolkit. A brief description of each tool and its purpose is shown in Table 8. In Part Two, an explanation of each tool is provided, along with guidelines for how and when to use the tools, and pitfalls to avoid. For an account of how the tools were derived, and an overview of the reasoning behind the tools, *see* Appendix E, pp.211–12.

Table 8. The intentional mentor's toolkit

TOOL #	NAME	DESCRIPTION
1	Purposeful communication	A relating and developing tool for achieving desired results in mentoring, based on listening, questioning and informing
2	Partnership	A connecting tool for engaging with the mentee for the duration of mentoring and linking the mentee to the broader community of practice
3	Goal-directed interaction	A progress tool for enhancing the mentee's success in setting and achieving goals, and realising their aspirational state of development
4	Curriculum and performance standards	A focusing tool for identifying competency and performance requirements relevant to the mentee's practice
5	Brief intervention (Tool #1, Purposeful communication with a focus on facilitation of desired outcomes within a short space of time)	An accelerating tool for helping the mentee overcome obstacles and accelerate their progress towards goal achievement
6	Resilience work (Tool #3, Goal-directed interaction with a focus on acquisition of sustained resilience)	A fortifying tool for engaging with the mentee in relation to impacts of work and how to turn stress into adaptation
7	Career guidance (Tool #3, Goal-directed interaction with a focus on career advancement)	A navigating tool for orienting the mentee towards useful resources, actions and decisions in relation to career
8	Confidentiality	A safety tool for protection of confidential information shared during mentoring
9	Evaluation	A discovery tool for identifying the mentee's response to mentoring and progress attributable to mentoring
10	Reflective practice of mentoring	A self-monitoring tool for learning about mentoring from experience

Reasons to apply I-Mentor with the Cycle of Caring and the intentional mentor's toolkit

By using I-Mentor with the Cycle of Caring and the intentional mentor's toolkit within your mentoring practice, you:

- perform the mentor's portion of the relational and developmental work of mentoring
- add structure to the mentoring partnership and process
- create a safe space for the mentee to access personalised assistance as they pursue developmental outcomes that are meaningful to them
- recognise and respond helpfully to the mentee's developmental needs for support, challenge and facilitation
- deliver support, challenge and facilitation in constructive and productive ways
- avoid any form of exploitation of the mentee or harm to the mentee
- have versatility as a mentor and are prepared for diverse mentoring scenarios (*see* Chapter 17, p.179)
- contribute to the mentee's development as a doctor in practice.

The case of Sam and Mikey

We illustrate the use of the toolkit with a mentoring case study involving Mikey, the consultant cardiologist from Chapter 2, p.23. We look back in time at Mikey's development as a medical registrar under the tutelage of his mentor Sam, a general physician. They appear briefly in each chapter of Part Two. They also appear in Chapter 16, p.139 within a case study that describes their mentoring partnership and process over time.

2

Part Two:
The intentional mentor's toolkit

5. Purposeful communication (Tool #1)

Case study: All of Sam's work as a mentor to Mikey was based on purposeful communication; communicating with results in mind. The results that both Sam and Mikey were seeking related to Mikey's development as a doctor. Sam was aware that as a mentor, there were three aspects to his role that were important to the success of mentoring: his work to build relationship, his work to foster development, and his way of structuring the mentoring partnership and process. He maintained his focus on pursuing results in these three areas, and used the elements of purposeful communication, listening, questioning and informing. Within each conversation with Mikey, Sam had a decision to make about the effects he wanted to have – to support, challenge and or facilitate – based on Mikey's needs. Again, listening, questioning and informing were the elements of his approach. Sam was acutely aware of the issue of bullying in medical training and was resolute about avoiding bullying in his partnership with Mikey, instead making his positive intentions clear through both verbal and non-verbal aspects of communication.

About the tool

Purposeful communication is the sending and receiving of both verbal and non-verbal messages with a result in mind. In medical practice, taking a medical history is an example of purposeful communication; there is a desired result (e.g. to make a diagnosis, or offer a therapeutic intervention), and the subsequent communication is structured around the desired result. In mentoring practice, having conversations that guide, inform, educate and inspire are all examples of purposeful communication. Listening, questioning and informing are the three elements of purposeful communication.

What it adds to the toolkit

Purposeful communication adds a **relating** and a **developing tool** to your toolkit. This tool is the mentor's 'universal tool' suitable for a wide range of uses, because relational work (work to build relationship) and developmental work (work to foster development) are the mainstays of mentoring practice. Purposeful communication is also necessary for delivering support, challenge and facilitation, types of influence you will exert as a mentor.

How to use the tool

Use active listening, questioning and informing to build relationship and foster development

Active listening is essential for purposes including understanding the mentee, demonstrating care, and cultivating partnership that is conducive to development. Questioning conveys interest in the mentee and their circumstances, and yields more information about the mentoring partnership, process and outcomes. A carefully crafted question may also help the mentee to make links in their own understanding of a situation or concept. Informing is imparting wisdom and experience; note that though this is vitally important, it is necessarily the third part of purposeful communication. Table 9 displays some of the many functions of listening, questioning and informing in terms of their relational and developmental purposes. Most doctors are familiar with the basics of listening, questioning and informing, so our focus in this chapter is on applications in mentoring. For a refresher on communication basics including listening, questioning and informing, *see* Appendix F, pp.213–14. For an overview of persuasive communication, *see* Appendix G, pp.215–17.

Table 9. Active listening, questioning and informing in relational and developmental work

ELEMENT OF COMMUNICATION	RELATIONAL WORK building relationship	DEVELOPMENTAL WORK fostering development
Active listening attending following reflecting (Kotzman, 1989)	Showing care, interest and availability\\Seeking to understand the mentee\\Noticing whether the mentee is engaging	Seeking to understand the mentee and the doctor they want to become\\Summarising and paraphrasing to confirm the mentee's message
Questioning objective questions reflective questions interpretive questions decisional questions (Spencer, 1989)	Showing interest and care\\Asking about the mentee's developmental needs\\Enquiring about what the mentee is experiencing	Asking the mentee to describe the doctor they want to become\\Prompting new understanding, insights and links between existing and new knowledge\\Exploring possibilities\\Discovering the mentee's goals and priorities\\Enquiring about barriers to performance

Informing	Stating availability and accessibility	Sharing experiences and resources
information about the mentee (feedback)	Describing commitment to the partnership	Explaining
information about oneself (self-disclosures)	Sharing experiences that are relevant to the mentee's situation	Encouraging
		Guiding
		Describing the next level of performance to strive for
information about medical practice	Acknowledging times of increased challenge for the mentee	Teaching
		Giving feedback
	Reassuring the mentee	
	Validating what the mentee is experiencing	

For examples of targets of developmental work, *see* Table 5, pp.43-44.

Listen actively

Listen actively to what the mentee is conveying, by attending, following and reflecting. This applies particularly in relation to what they are conveying about the types of support, challenge and facilitation they need from you in service of their goals. Incongruence between the mentee's verbal and non-verbal messages may point to inner conflict or difficulties that need attention.

Question

Medical students are taught intensively about using two categories of questions, open and closed. Open questions invite detailed, lengthy answers and closed questions elicit short, direct answers. The focused conversation method makes use of four categories of questions (Spencer, 1989), with high utility in mentoring.

- *Objective questions* to elicit data, facts and sensory information, for example: "What did you hear your boss say?"
- *Reflective questions* to elicit personal reactions and associations, for example: "What is it about the situation that distressed you?"
- *Interpretive questions* to elicit meaning, significance and implications, for example: "What is the significance of the situation to you?"
- *Decisional questions* to elicit resolutions for the future, for example: "How will you respond to similar situations in the future?"

Asking the right question is particularly important. This is one of the basic tenets of a medical history, and it is similarly important in mentoring. It is through questions that we recognise underlying motives, values and worldviews. For example, most people do not have at the front of conscious thought why they might become distressed if their boss is not happy with their work. This is a very reasonable response, but one that may come from different places for different people. For some it may come from the clinical sphere "I want the patient to get the best care, and I didn't deliver that today." For others it may be the professional sphere, "I'm now going to find it very awkward to work with this person." For others it might be a concern over career "I wanted that boss to be a reference to get onto program x, and I'm worried I've lost his/her respect." Others might have their whole self-worth tied up in being a good doctor, and it is a crushing experience when they do not do it well. Usually it is a combination. The correctly framed question can help bring clarity and subsequently help set a goal to improve.

Appreciative enquiry uses positive, strengths-focused questions to explore concerns and aspirations in affirmative ways, with the aim of bringing about more of what is already working well, and generating new possibilities and innovations (Cooperrider, Whitney & Stavros, 2008; Stratton-Berkessel, 2010). Note the contrast to traditional problem solving methods which begin with a defined problem and cause analysis, as shown in Table 10. Exploring the mentee's aspirational state of development is an example of envisioning what might be.

Table 10. Contrasting a traditional problem solving approach and the Appreciative Inquiry approach

PROBLEM SOLVING	APPRECIATIVE INQUIRY
Identifying a problem	Appreciating the best of 'what is' in terms of peak experiences, strengths, assets and successes (discover)
Analysing causes of the problem	Imagining 'what might be' based on past successes, current strengths and possibilities (dream)
Analysing possible solutions to the problem	Discussing 'what should be' in terms of design elements for manifesting the dream (design)
Action planning	Innovating 'what will be' by reinforcing and rewarding continuous adaptation, using the discovery, dream and design stages

Source: Cooperrider, Whitney & Stavros (2008); Stratton-Berkessel (2010)

Questioning is an art with potentially powerful effects. Vogt, Brown and Isaccs (2003) explain how to craft questions that catalyse insight, innovation and action. This knowledge is relevant to crafting powerful questions in your work with the mentee, and for teaching the mentee to craft their own powerful questions in their everyday practice and during reflective enquiry.

Inform

Three broad categories of information you might offer as a mentor are information about the mentee (e.g. feedback on performance), yourself (e.g. self-disclosures), and medical practice (e.g. best practice). In keeping with the adult learning principles of Knowles (1984), information you provide should:

- give the mentee choice in what is discussed, and the responsibility for their own learning
- build on the mentee's existing knowledge and skills
- connect to the mentee's roles and tasks
- be useful now
- connect with and stimulate the mentee's interests (*see* Appendix H, pp.219–23 for guides to applying adult learning principles).

Information that is clear, concise, concrete, correct, coherent, complete and courteous, known as the 7 Cs of communication (Cutlip & Center, 1952), can help your message to reach the mentee.

Use active listening, questioning and informing to support, challenge and facilitate

The elements of purposeful communication, active listening, questioning and informing, are also the vehicle for delivering support, challenge and facilitation in service of the mentee's goals. Table 11 gives examples of how you might use active listening, questioning and informing to support, challenge and facilitate.

Table 11. Using active listening, questioning and informing to support, challenge and facilitate

EFFECT	ELEMENT OF COMMUNICATION		
	ACTIVE LISTENING	QUESTIONING	INFORMING
Support (strengthening)	Listening to gain an understanding of the mentee's challenges and struggles, personal coping strategies, and perceived resources Listening to convey care and demonstrate that the mentee is not alone in facing challenges	Asking questions to explore the mentee's challenges and struggles, personal coping strategies, and perceived resources	Informing the mentee of available resources Providing validation, reassurance and encouragement
Challenge (inducing helpful strain)	Listening to gain an understanding of the mentee's situation, aspirational state of development and goals	Asking questions to explore the mentee's situation, aspirational state of development and goals Asking difficult questions	Informing the mentee of aspects of essential tasks that were performed well, and aspects that were overlooked or that need improvement Describing the next level of performance to pursue
Facilitation (enabling breakthrough)	Listening to gain an understanding of barriers to the mentee's goal achievement	Asking questions to guide reflective enquiry Assisting the mentee to form their own reflective enquiry questions	Providing the mentee with information relevant to overcoming obstacles and making progress in pursuit of their goals

Use agreed channels for communicating

Given that communication is essential for the quality of the relational and developmental work of mentoring, it is important to establish upfront an understanding of how and when communication will occur during the course of mentoring. An initial partnership discussion is an opportunity to have this discussion and form an agreement about communicating in comfortable and effective ways. The agreement might include acceptable methods of communicating, places for communicating, the timing of conversations, off-limits times for communicating, the frequency of contact, the turnaround time for a response to communication, and more.

Contemporary options for communicating using technology mean that mentoring can easily occur across different locations. However, communication tends to be more effective in person (e.g. it offers more options for interacting, such as the use of demonstrations, and for picking up on the nuances of the exchange), and face-to-face meetings should occur at times, if possible.

Be constructive

Whatever combination of listening, questioning and informing that you use to communicate with the mentee, ensure it is constructive. Previous chapters have highlighted the importance of the quality of support, challenge and facilitation in mentoring. Especially significant is the quality of challenge. A fine line exists between constructive challenge necessary for growth and development, and destructive challenge. The zone of constructive communication is highlighted in Figure 12.

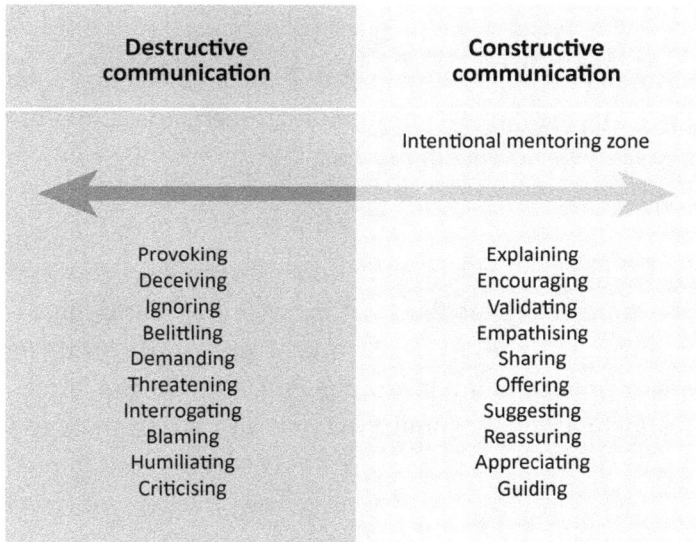

Destructive communication	Constructive communication
	Intentional mentoring zone
←	→
Provoking	Explaining
Deceiving	Encouraging
Ignoring	Validating
Belittling	Empathising
Demanding	Sharing
Threatening	Offering
Interrogating	Suggesting
Blaming	Reassuring
Humiliating	Appreciating
Criticising	Guiding

Figure 12. The destructive-constructive communication spectrum

Question constructively

While questioning serves so many constructive functions, it is also commonly used in the practice of 'teaching by humiliation' (Scott, Caldwell, Barnes & Barrett, 2015). As most readers will have experienced, at times a question can be asked (often in a group setting) with an aggressive agenda designed not to probe for areas that require development, but rather to induce a sense of fear, shame or inferiority. There is a false belief that this kind of questioning will create such a fear of getting the wrong answer that the learner will study extra hard to avoid further humiliation. This kind of questioning is fundamentally destructive, and is entirely counter to the ethos of intentional mentoring.

Constructive questioning serves two educational purposes. Firstly, it helps the mentor know the mentee's baseline knowledge; to pitch the teaching at the most appropriate level. Secondly, recalling information helps to reinforce learned knowledge, and so the act of answering a question helps to consolidate the mentee's knowledge. Constructive questioning begins with broad, conceptual questions, and eventually narrows down to more difficult, niche questions to find a teachable point. It is important that the mentor maintains a gentle, calm and non-judgmental demeanour that encourages participation.

Give constructive feedback

Feedback is "information that a system uses to make adjustments in reaching a goal" (Ende, 1983, p.777). In the context of mentoring, feedback is information that the mentee uses to make adjustments in reaching their mentoring goals, including work performance goals.

Murphy et al. (2012) use the term insightful practice to describe doctors' willingness to receive and act on credible feedback to improve their performance. The process involves the doctor accepting responsibility and accountability for their performance, accessing a suite of independent feedback, reflecting on the evidence gathered, setting objectives for performance improvement, and taking steps to improve their performance.

The importance of credible feedback to performance improvement is underscored by the work of Dunning, Johnson, Ehrlinger and Kruger (2003) whose research on awareness of incompetence suggests that "in many social and intellectual domains, people are unaware of their incompetence, innocent of their ignorance" and "where they lack skill or knowledge, they greatly overestimate their expertise and talent" (p.83).

One of the most appealing aspects of mentoring for the mentee is the opportunity to access feedback without fear of retribution or an insensitive response. The mentor's commitment to constructiveness in relational work assures the mentee a safe space for exploring their work performance, and receiving constructive feedback that they can action.

Receiving constructive feedback:

- contributes to insight
- improves motivation to change
- drives learning and performance improvement
- narrows the gap between actual and desired performance
- enables achievement of performance goals.

Conversely, a lack of constructive feedback can result in:

- trial and error at the patient's expense
- continuation of poor performance
- a missed opportunity for better performance
- good performance not being reinforced.

When delivered poorly, feedback can lead to defensiveness, embarrassment, humiliation and demoralisation. Many frameworks for delivering constructive feedback have been developed from the seminal work of Ende (1983), who stated that feedback should:

- be undertaken with the teacher and trainee working as allies with common goals
- be well-timed and expected
- be based on first-hand data
- be regulated in quantity and limited to behaviours that are remediable
- be phrased in descriptive and non-evaluative language
- deal with specific performances, not generalisations
- offer subjective data, labelled as such
- deal with decisions and actions, rather than assumed intentions or interpretations.

Debriefing with good judgment is an approach to giving feedback that is carefully crafted to serve the purpose of reinforcing desired practices while discouraging unhelpful practices. It is delivered sensitively and with clearly articulated frames of reference for the feedback (Rudolph, Simon, Rivard, Dufresne & Raemer, 2007; Rudolph, Simon, Raemer & Eppich, 2008).

See Appendix H, pp.222–4 and Appendix I, p.226 for guides to delivering constructive feedback.

Take care with tone

In conversation with the mentee, your tone of voice reveals your attitudes, and has the potential to affect how the mentee feels about engaging with you in the mentoring partnership and process. Considering your normal tone of voice, how would a reasonable person feel in conversation with you? Do you convey care through tone? Constructive feedback may be interpreted by the mentee as harsh criticism if the tone is harsh, and this may demoralise rather than empower them to change. An effective surgical mentor we know raises the matter of tone upfront with his mentees. He tells them in advance that when they call him at work he will probably come across as terse because of the intensity of his work, but he is interested in talking with them and is willing to make a time to talk later.

When to use purposeful communication

This tool is for **all** sessions.

As a mentor, your work is two-fold, to build relationship and to foster development, including delivery of support, challenge and facilitation as required by the mentee. Purposeful communication is used for this work throughout mentoring.

Of course, using purposeful communication does not mean that you relate to the mentee in a robotic way, or that all of your communication is business-like. Indeed, the best mentoring partnerships are the ones that have an organic flavour, where there is some personal buy-in and easy conversation. However, the primary purpose of intentional mentoring relates to the pursuit of developmental outcomes that are meaningful to the mentee and your communications should be used to this end.

Pitfalls to avoid

- Poor listening e.g. not listening enough
- Poor questioning e.g. questioning aggressively, excessively, or with the intent to humiliate
- Poor informing e.g. providing irrelevant information, excessive information or unhelpful feedback
- Overusing self-disclosure

- Overdoing developmental work at the expense of relational work
- Making assumptions about what the mentee wants to focus on in a session, and the kinds of support, challenge and facilitation they require
- Giving solutions to a problem without letting the mentee experience the struggle towards breakthrough

Case study

To find out how Sam used this tool with Mikey during a mentoring session, turn to:

- Conversation – Partnership set-up, *see* pp.140–3
- Conversation – Learning knowledge, *see* pp.144–7
- Conversation – Learning a skill, *see* pp.148–51
- Conversation – Understanding and addressing performance problems that are complex, *see* pp.166–9

6. Partnership (Tool #2)

Case study: Sam and Mikey met through a formal mentoring program. Their decision to form a mentoring partnership was based upon their shared specialty (general medicine) and shared interests (cycling and golf). As the partnership developed, it became foundational to Mikey's transition from an inexperienced, new medical registrar into a capable and competent medical registrar. An aspect of Sam and Mikey's partnership was the natural chemistry of their relationship. They developed a camaraderie, which made the mentoring partnership a more authentic experience and helped to develop trust.

About the tool

A partnership is an alliance of two or more people deciding to work together on the same cause. The decision to work together may be based on a superficial bond created by an agreement or a deeper bond created by heartfelt commitment to a cause.

What it adds to the toolkit

Partnership adds a **connecting tool** to your toolkit. The connection between the mentor and the mentee serves as a channel for the mentee to access the mentor's expertise and to receive beneficial support, challenge and facilitation. The connection between the mentor and the mentee also links the mentee to the broader community of practice and the abundance of resources it contains.

Many successful mentoring partnerships have an organic component growing out of an existing friendship or acquaintance, or the natural chemistry of human relationships, but those dynamics are not essential. A mentoring partnership can emerge from the decision of the mentor and the mentee to work together with the same purpose in mind, that is, the development of the mentee.

How to use the tool

Notice opportunities for forming a mentoring partnership

Opportunities for forming a mentoring partnership exist wherever there is a junior medical colleague who is willing to receive assistance from a senior, and a senior medical colleague who is willing to give assistance to a junior. An enquiry is often the catalyst for a mentoring partnership to begin to form, for example:

- A junior medical colleague seeks out your assistance and enquires about your availability to be a mentor
- A peer or a mentoring program coordinator enquires about your availability as a mentor, on behalf of a junior medical colleague
- A junior medical colleague shows potential, or experiences problems, in an area of practice, and you offer them assistance

Often the starting point for mentoring is not so obvious or deliberate, and mentoring simply evolves from an existing relationship, for example:

- Corridor conversations with a junior medical colleague turn into regular discussions about challenges of practice
- A junior medical colleague seeks your guidance on one issue and returns for guidance on a broader set of issues over time
- A trainee asks to continue to access your assistance and guidance after a clinical placement has concluded

Be aware of what you bring to mentoring

As a mentor you have the potential to be a highly positive influence on the mentee. To be the most constructive and productive contributor to mentoring that you can be (and avoid being a destructive influence on the mentee), consider the following aspects of what you bring to mentoring, prior to engaging in a mentoring partnership:

- A vision of the mentor you want to become
- Your intentions as a mentor
- The style of mentoring you would like to offer; a way of engaging with mentees that feels natural and appropriate to you
- Your attitudes towards learners and novices, and your expectations of them
- Your past experiences as a doctor and a mentor that you can draw from for the benefit of the mentee

- Your willingness to explore new opportunities and experiences
- Areas of strength in your practice as a doctor and in your work assisting junior medical colleagues to develop
- Limitations in your practice as a doctor and in your work assisting junior medical colleagues to develop
- The mentoring knowledge and or skills your need to develop further to be an effective mentor
- Your availability to help junior medical colleagues to develop
- Your energy for the developmental and relational work of mentoring and the number of mentees you could comfortably work with

See Appendix K, pp.231–6 for a resource designed to assist you with this reflection in preparation for your role as an intentional mentor.

Apply the Cycle of Caring

The Cycle of Caring stages of empathic attachment, active involvement and felt separation (Skovholt, 2005), *see* Chapter 4, pp.52–3, are landmarks for the mentor during the course of mentoring. They give the mentor reference points for where they are now and where they will go next on the mentee's developmental journey, and what is required from them in each moment. The three stages frame everything that happens during mentoring, for example, the following processes.

Form a partnership using empathic attachment

Create a safe space

Staging of the partnership matters; relational work must begin before developmental work begins, to create a safe, supportive and nurturing developmental space. Too much questioning or challenging without a trusting relationship in place can feel unsafe to mentees, so if the partnership is new, be aware that you are in the empathic attachment stage and build relationship and trust as a priority.

Creating a safe space involves conveying acceptance of the mentee just the way they are; as an individual with strengths, weaknesses and vulnerabilities. The words that you use to reassure them that they are safe to talk, and accepted as they are, can allow a collaborative partnership to flourish. Sharing personally (if you are comfortable with this) can help to model and build trust, and create a safe space.

Choosing a suitable location and surroundings also helps. A neutral area where both mentor and mentee are comfortable, such as a café, can be conducive to building partnership. Some mentees prefer to participate in mentoring in private settings at times, so check with them before making arrangements.

Early in the partnership, setting aside time outside of work for a discussion or activity (e.g. finding a common interest over coffee or lunch) can make the subsequent mentoring experience easier.

Reach a shared understanding of mentoring

Given the variety of perspectives on mentoring, it is worthwhile to have a conversation early in the partnership about what mentoring means for you both. This might include clarifying that mentoring is a partnership, that both mentor and mentee have responsibilities to fulfil, and that commitment and effort are required for the duration of mentoring in order to achieve desired outcomes.

Identify the mentee's initial mentoring goals and anticipated developmental needs

What has prompted the mentee to be involved in mentoring? The mentee is likely to have an idea about what they want to get out of mentoring. Usually they will have decided, "I want Dr X to mentor me because she's a great surgeon and I want to be a great surgeon too" or "I want Dr Y to mentor me because I'm really struggling to cope and I think he would be understanding and helpful." Explore the mentee's motivations to engage in the mentoring partnership and process, and their ideas about the resources and experiences they anticipate they will need in order to develop in ways that are relevant to their job, career path and aspirations in the medical profession.

Decide on collaboration

After gathering information about the mentee's initial mentoring goals and anticipated developmental needs, you are in a position to assess your suitability as a mentor to the mentee. Is there a match between what the mentee is seeking in the way of support, challenge and facilitation, and what you are willing to offer? Are there any foreseeable barriers to a successful mentoring partnership with the mentee? Is there another mentor who might be significantly more helpful to the mentee? These are all considerations. If you are unsure about the suitability of the partnership, consider forming a mentoring partnership for a trial period. Also consider your existing mentoring commitments and agree to work with a manageable number of mentees. Three mentees in a formal capacity is probably enough, considering the other mentoring activities you will be involved in during your day to day work.

Occasionally, a potential mentoring partnership may involve a mentee who you are expected to formally assess as part of another role, for example, a supervisory role. Adding formal assessment to a mentoring partnership can be tricky, and it may have detrimental effects on the mentoring partnership (particularly if the mentee does not perform to an appropriate level). Of course, the other side of this is that the mentor is well-positioned to identify where the mentee needs to improve in order to be deemed competent through formal assessment. Realistically, most assessment that occurs at the supervisor-trainee level is formative rather than summative, and concerns about a potential conflict of interest can be overcome with transparent communication. Infrequently, it may be necessary to either conclude the mentoring partnership or transfer the mentee to another supervisor if a conflict of interest arises and cannot be resolved. If a conflict of interest is likely, it is advisable to avoid the dual relationship from the outset. *See* Chapter 17, p.181–2 for an overview of the role of the supervisor who acts as a mentor.

Discuss expectations for the partnership

After deciding to collaborate, the next step is to discuss expectations. This includes expectations about the mentee's initial goals, the developmental needs that you will aim to address in mentoring, the frequency and methods of contact, boundaries including off-limits times and places, the anticipated course and duration of the partnership, confidentiality and privacy, and the scope of information sharing, for example what you both do and do not need to know about each other's activities. Discussions of expectations should also include responsibilities that you will both take on. If you expect the mentee to achieve as much as possible independently before seeking your guidance, articulate this up front.

A reality of mentoring is that the partnership will evolve from the very beginning, in expected and unexpected ways. At times the dynamic of the partnership may be easy and comfortable, and at times it may be tense and uncomfortable. This does not necessarily mean that the mentoring partnership is unsuitable; all close relationships have positive and negative aspects (Eby, 2012). Be open to this, and honest about it in your early discussions with the mentee.

Establish an agreement

Of the expectations you discuss, some will be particularly important to building and maintaining a partnership; these should form the basis of an agreement. Your agreement can be formalised as a written agreement, or it can simply be a verbal agreement. Written agreements can be experienced as too formal. Verbal agreements in our experience are more applicable and helpful. Sometimes working out agreements can feel a little bit awkward and contrived. However, it can be useful to ensure that unspoken assumptions are articulated, so you both can be clear about your expectations. Even so, not everything needs to be articulated at the start. It should not feel like a business contract.

Figure 13 highlights some of the areas that may be important to establish from the outset and to include in your mentoring agreement, whether in verbal or written form. *See* Appendix K, pp.239–40 for a mentoring agreement template and a checklist to guide an initial partnership discussion.

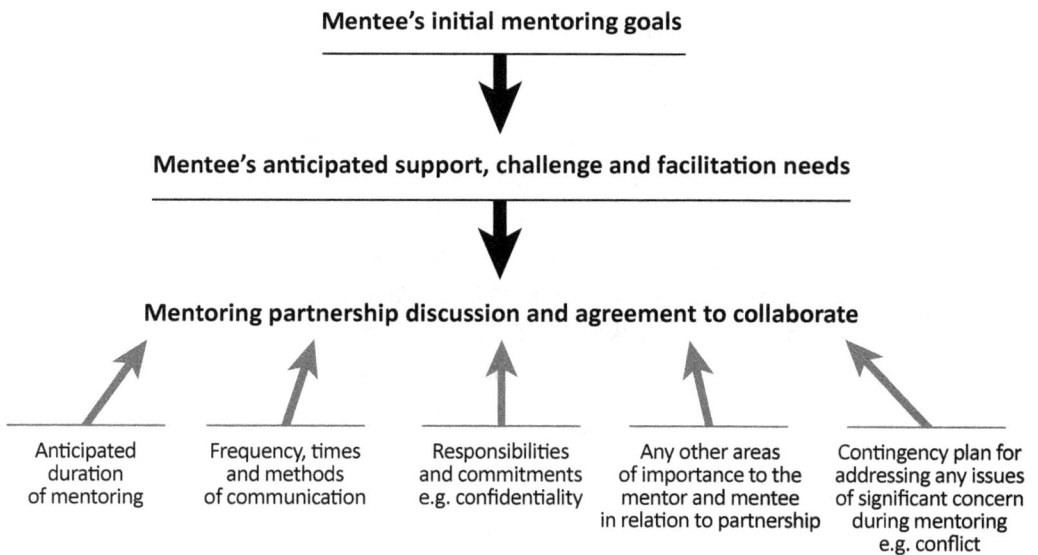

Mentee's initial mentoring goals

Mentee's anticipated support, challenge and facilitation needs

Mentoring partnership discussion and agreement to collaborate

| Anticipated duration of mentoring | Frequency, times and methods of communication | Responsibilities and commitments e.g. confidentiality | Any other areas of importance to the mentor and mentee in relation to partnership | Contingency plan for addressing any issues of significant concern during mentoring e.g. conflict |

Figure 13. Components of a mentoring agreement

Prepare the mentee

The mentee may benefit from self-awareness activities and reflective enquiry in preparation for mentoring. For example, a mentee who is a junior doctor could review the curriculum standards applicable to their stage of training to identify areas to focus on during mentoring. *See* Appendix K, pp.237–8 for a resource containing sample questions organised by categories of the Australian Curriculum Framework for Junior Doctors (Confederation of Postgraduate Medical Education Councils, 2012).

Collaborate using active involvement

Perform your mentor role

Your role is to do relational and developmental work with the mentee, incorporating support, challenge and facilitation, and to add structure to the mentoring as described in Chapter 4, pp.41–9 and Appendix D, pp.205–7. While performing your mentor role, keep the focus on the mentee advancing towards their aspirational state of development. At times the mentee's aspirational state of development will need to be adjusted, for example, if they change their career path, or realise their original aspirational state of development and form another.

Re-negotiate the partnership at intervals

As illustrated in the Model of Intentional Mentoring (*see* pp.12–13), mentoring involves a feedback loop: relational work affects developmental work, and vice versa. As the mentee develops (or circumstances change), the partnership is likely to change too. For example, the mentee may initially seek help with improving their resume to get onto a training program, and after achieving this goal they set a new goal related to preparing for post-graduate exams whilst working and managing a family. The partnership agreement should be renegotiated at intervals to ensure that there is still a match between what the mentee is seeking in the way of support, challenge and facilitation, and what the mentor is willing to offer.

Renegotiation of the partnership is also due if mentoring sessions or activities are not happening as agreed. This can be a time of exploring obstacles to participation, how the mentor and mentee might be contributing to this result, and what needs to change for mentoring to proceed as planned.

Part ways when the time is right, using felt separation

Parting ways is a normal and natural part of mentoring because mentoring is intended to be a transitional developmental partnership and process. 'When the time is right' encompasses many different scenarios, for example:

- when the desired outcomes have been achieved
- when mentoring is evolving into a friendship and it would be useful to conclude the partnership and redefine it as a friendship with a new set of expectations attached
- when you are unable to meet any of the mentee's developmental needs
- when things are not going well.

Both mentor and mentee should be involved in the decision to change the nature of the mentoring or part ways. When a mentoring partnership is about conclude or transition into another type of relationship, felt separation, that is giving importance to separating in a felt and meaningful way, is a way to end the partnership well (Skovholt, 2005).

When to use partnership

This tool is for **all** sessions.

As a fundamental part of mentoring, partnership is ongoing for the duration of mentoring. Pay attention to the quality of the partnership at all times and give as much attention to relational work as developmental work.

Pitfalls to avoid

- Engaging in mentoring at the request of a third party (e.g. a supervisor) who expects to be informed of the details of the work undertaken
- Deciding for the mentee what they should work on during the course of mentoring
- Agreeing to form mentoring partnerships with too many mentees
- Allowing a partnership of unhealthy dependency to form
- Unintentionally breaching the professional boundaries of the partnership

- Failing to re-negotiate the partnership as the mentee develops or as circumstances change
- Not having a contingency plan for addressing any issues of significant concern during mentoring e.g. conflict

Case study

To find out how Sam used this tool with Mikey during a mentoring session, turn to:

- Conversation – Partnership set-up, *see* pp.140–3
- Conversation – Learning a skill, *see* pp.148–51
- Conversation – Concluding mentoring, *see* pp.173–8

7. Goal-Directed Interaction (Tool #3)

Case study: One of Sam's sayings as he worked with Mikey was 'Where are you at now, and where do you want to be?' During his interactions with Mikey, Sam gave importance to Mikey's goals, and ensured their collaborative efforts were organised around Mikey's goals.

About the tool

A goal is the object of a person's ambition, a desired result. Goal-directed interaction is interaction that places one or more goals in focus, and uses the goal/s as a reference point for all collaborative efforts. Another way of thinking about goal-directed interaction is interaction in service of goal achievement.

What it adds to the toolkit

Goal-directed interaction adds a **progress tool** to your toolkit. As a unit of the developmental work of mentoring, goal-directed interaction ideally enhances the mentee's success at goal setting and achievement, and progress towards their aspirational state of development. Goals may relate to knowing (e.g. acquiring knowledge, skills and competencies), doing (e.g. accessing opportunities for participation and overcoming barriers to performance) or being (e.g. recognising and enacting values in practice). The interaction is not limited to any particular activities in the pursuit of goal achievement. As long as a goal is in sight and the activities are designed to lead towards goal achievement, goal-directed interaction is occurring.

Goal-directed interaction is also relevant to the relational work of mentoring, for example, goals related to building a partnership, forming a mentoring agreement, re-negotiating the agreement, or concluding mentoring.

How to use the tool

Assist the mentee to set goals

Explore the mentee's aspirational state of development

The ultimate aim of goal-directed interaction is progress by the mentee, towards or to their aspirational state of development. At the start of mentoring, the mentee may be unaware of their aspirational state of development and may need your assistance with formulating one. Asking the mentee to describe their aspirational state of development is similar to asking them to describe the doctor they wish to become. The exercise requires the mentee to imagine and describe their ideal repertoire of knowing, doing, and being in the medical profession and ideally includes reflection on strengths to capitalise on and weaknesses to address. As explained in Chapter 1, p.10 the aspirational state of development is relatively stable but not static, and serves as goal posts for developmental work for a time.

The mentee's job description, containing a description of knowledge, behaviours and values associated with their role, can be a useful starting point for this exercise. However, a static job description does not capture the unique and changing characteristics of the work environment, and does not equate to the way the mentee experiences work within their organisation. The curriculum applicable to the mentee's stage of training, containing an overview of requisite knowledge, behaviours and values, can also be a useful starting point. However, a curriculum does not contain information about the mentee's individual interests, or factor in whether they want to be conservative or aggressive in treating disease, or primarily academic with research interests, or a head of unit involved in administration and leadership roles, to name a few examples.

While a job description or curriculum may be the basis of the mentee's aspirational state of development, these documents are no substitute for an aspirational state of development that factors in the mentee's mandated and chosen aspirations. Encourage the mentee to personalise their aspirational state of development beyond wanting to become a specialist who can do all the things on the curriculum, or aspiring to be a doctor who fulfils the requirements of their job description. The incredible breadth of options available to doctors is both a great opportunity and a challenge to work with. As a mentor you are in a position to help the mentee to recognise and move towards or realise their aspirational state of development. *See* Appendix K, pp.242–4 for a worksheet designed to assist the mentee with this exercise.

Identify goals relevant to the mentee's aspirational state of development

With an aspirational state of development in mind, the mentee is ready to translate their aspirational state of development to learning, performance and values-related goals, as shown in Figure 14. The mentee's goals may relate to becoming more, for example, becoming more involved, skilled, functional at higher levels of difficulty, consistent, efficient, adaptive to non-routine situations, compliant with regulations, or aware of thinking. The mentee's goals may also relate to becoming less, for example, becoming less error prone, formulaic and uncomfortable with uncertainty. Often mentees will not know where to start in setting goals, particularly new interns, and will require guidance. In the early, overwhelming time of transition to the workforce, their goals may simply relate to getting comfortable in the job, gaining reassurance about work performance, and making time for activities outside work.

Figure 14. Translating the mentee's aspirational state of development to goals

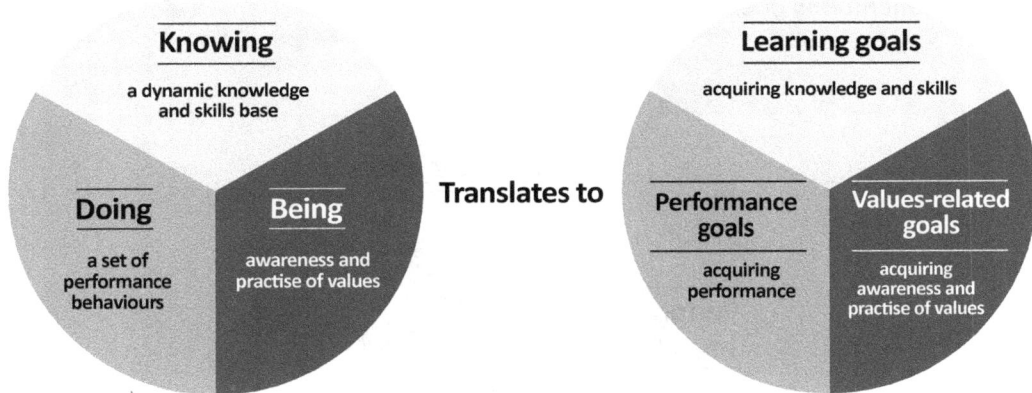

Knowing
a dynamic knowledge and skills base

Doing
a set of performance behaviours

Being
awareness and practise of values

Translates to

Learning goals
acquiring knowledge and skills

Performance goals
acquiring performance

Values-related goals
acquiring awareness and practise of values

Commonly, mentees' priorities for development fall into roughly four categories, clinical skills and knowledge, professionalism and teamwork, resilience and career advancement. Some mentees may develop career advancement goals at the expense of the other goal areas because they are career-focused. However, this may be detrimental to the career goal itself. For example, an intern we know was so focused on becoming a neurosurgeon that she neglected her clinical duties in favour of doing research. This lead to poor clinical development subsequently hindering her progress through internship and hence her career path. The mentee is not necessarily going to know what issues they are likely to face and may benefit from developing goals in all four categories over the course of mentoring. Additionally, categories may interact with each other, for example, a serious clinical problem such as a clinically significant error can affect well-being (and vice versa), and resolution in one area may depend on resolution in another.

Delineate a subset of goals that the mentee would like to work on in mentoring

The mentee may have a range of goals in mind for moving towards or realising their aspirational state of development. You do not have to attempt to help the mentee with every goal they wish to set and achieve. The mentee should be a participant in a range of doctor development strategies and have a range of doctors (e.g. supervisors and educators) helping them to set and achieve goals. Select a manageable number of mentoring goals considering goals the partnership is best equipped to achieve, as shown in Figure 15. With mentoring goals selected, a plan for goal achievement can be formed.

Figure 15. Selecting mentoring goals

Translate mentoring goals to SMART goals

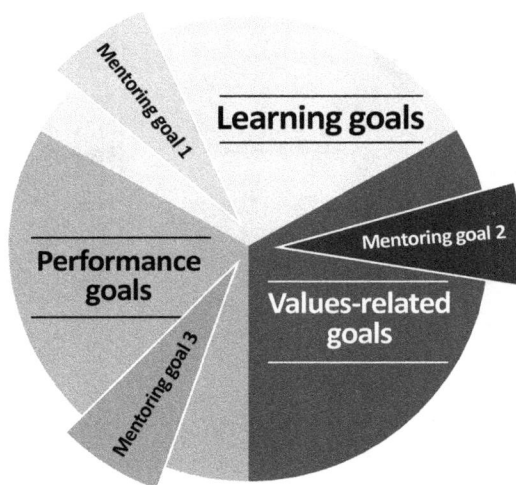

An initial discussion of proposed goals takes place during the partnership set-up meeting. At subsequent meetings, goals are decided and refined to SMART goals as part of planning for goal achievement. SMART is an acronym that frames a statement of results to be achieved, based on the following criteria.

- Specific: targets a specific area for improvement,
- Measurable: the result can be checked against a benchmark,
- Assignable: the contributors to goal achievement are identified,
- Realistic: results are achievable with the available resources; the goal is appropriate for the individual given their level of knowledge, skills and resources, or can be achieved through breaking the goal down into smaller, achievable sub-goals,
- Time related: a time frame is specified for the achievement of the goal (Doran, 1981; Haughey, 2014).

Table 12 displays the five components of SMART goals and sample questions that can be used as part of the process. If the SMART approach feels too structured for the mentee, it can be adapted to suit the individual.

Table 12. SMART goal setting

GOAL COMPONENT	SAMPLE QUESTIONS
Specific	What result would you like to achieve? How does the goal relate to your aspirational state of development and what you want to know, do and be in the medical profession?
Measurable	How will you know you have achieved the result?
Assignable	Who will participate in the pursuit of goal achievement? What will they contribute?
Realistic	What knowledge, skills and resources give you confidence that you can achieve the goal?
Time related	What is your timeframe for achieving the goal?

Assist the mentee to achieve their goals

Invite the mentee to choose the agenda for the session

The mentee may have a number of mentoring goals. An informal session agenda gives priority to one or more of those goals. The mentee is likely to be more receptive to mentoring if they are given the opportunity to choose the agenda for the session. If you think that their agenda is in service of avoidance, rather than in service of their goals, you have the option of querying and gently challenging them about their choice of agenda.

Identify what the mentee needs from you in service of their goals

With the session agenda decided and one or more goals in mind, ascertain what the mentee needs from you in terms of support, challenge and facilitation, to pursue goal achievement. Consider whether the four sources of information about need (felt, normative, expressed and comparative needs, as described in Chapter 3, pp.38–9), might apply to the mentee's goals. For example:

1. *Felt need.* What support, challenge or facilitation is the mentee asking for from you, in order to achieve their goals?
2. *Normative need.* What does an authority expect the mentee to need in terms of support, challenge and facilitation, to achieve their goals?
3. *Comparative need.* Based on the needs of similar doctors, what can be assumed about the mentee's needs for support, challenge and facilitation?
4. *Expressed need.* Based on other doctors' uptake of services or resources, what can be inferred about the mentee's needs for support, challenge and facilitation?

The mentee will not always be able to verbalise their felt needs in terms of the need for support, challenge and facilitation. For example, they may not explicitly state that they need your support. They are more likely to describe a situation, problem or opportunity they are experiencing and convey that they would like guidance in seeking a resolution. In relation to developing knowledge and skills, the conscious competence learning model (Broadwell, 1969) suggests that doctors move through stages of awareness of their competence, and at earlier stages, they don't know what they don't know. This makes it especially important for you to be able to recognise the mentee's needs from other perspectives. The mentee's needs will change throughout the course of mentoring and as such needs analysis will be a continuous process.

How far will you go in addressing the mentee's needs for support, challenge and facilitation? This is an area where balance is required; finding the balance between helping in a way that makes a difference and allowing the mentee to retain a reasonable level of independence. Identifying the extent to which meeting developmental needs is in the mentee's best interests is a matter of judgment. This may require you to occasionally say no to requests for assistance.

Participate in activities in service of the mentee's goals

The intentional mentoring process is similar to action research, where action occurs, and effects are observed to inform the next action. Choose activities based on the likelihood of leading to the desired outcome (goal achievement), using the criteria of feasibility, plausibility and testability. Feasibility refers to whether the activity can realistically lead to goal achievement. Plausibility refers to the logic of the pathway and whether the steps are in the right order for goal achievement. Testability refers to whether it is possible to measure the contribution of the activity to goal achievement (Aspen Institute, 1997). There are often many paths to goal achievement, just as there are many routes to a destination.

On the path to goal achievement, let the mentee feel their way. The metaphor of curling is useful here. Curling is a sport played on an ice ring where players push a heavy disk down towards a mark (like lawn bowls on ice). Two players rough up the ice with broom-like objects in front of the disk to slow it down, speed it up, and or change its direction slightly. The mentor is much more like the player who roughs up the ice than the player who pushes the disk down. Mentors do not set people on their path. Instead they help make small adjustments and refinements to help them land in the right spot.

Activities may be conversation-based, action-based, or both. Common activities include:

- formulating an aspirational state of development
- discussing goals and plans
- exploring options
- collaborative problem solving and decision making
- sharing experiences
- teaching and learning
- deliberate practice with coaching (*see* Appendix A, pp.193–4)
- simulation and debriefing
- giving and receiving feedback
- demonstrations and verbalisation of thinking/thinking aloud
- guided reflective enquiry
- referral
- recognising and celebrating achievements.

Cervero and Gaines (2015) state that greater improvement in physician performance and patient health is achieved through continuing medical education activities that are more interactive, use more methods, involve multiple exposures, are longer, and are focused on outcomes that are considered important by physicians. Activities with these features are typical of mentoring activities.

In between sessions and encounters, the mentee is responsible for carrying out further tasks related to goal achievement, such as practising skills learnt during mentoring, acquiring additional knowledge, researching, focusing, journaling and reflecting. If the groundwork for the partnership is appropriately laid, you can usually have brief but effective follow-ups. There are many ways and locations to do follow-ups, for example in clinical scenarios, during corridor conversations, and in the tea room.

Address incongruence in the mentee's aspirational state of development, goals and actions

During the course of mentoring you may notice incongruence in the mentee's aspirational state of development and set of goals, or incongruence in their goals and actions. This incongruence can be an indicator of goals that are not relevant or realistically achievable, even if the mentee is dedicated, driven and focused on achievement. For example, a mentee may want to become a surgeon, get married and have five children, all within the space of five years. By examining incongruence in a curious and gentle way, goals can be adjusted to be more realistic, or additional planning and problem solving can take place to increase the likelihood of goal achievement.

Be guided by the mentee on the amount of structure to the interaction

An interaction may be heavily structured, completely unstructured, or somewhere in between. Be guided by the mentee on the amount of structure you add to the interaction. This is something that you and the mentee can experiment with, or discuss and decide on upfront. A benefit of structuring a session is that you can make sure you cover the most important topics, such as whether the mentee has carried out tasks set for completion between sessions. Keep in mind that some mentees prefer a casual, natural conversation rather than working through a checklist of items, and some mentees will not respond well to a formal structure as they may feel they are being assessed.

At the final session, part ways positively

The primary goal of the final session is ending the partnership positively and moving on separately. This session provides an opportunity for felt separation; acknowledging what took place over the course of mentoring, what the benefits and effects of mentoring were, and what resources the mentee acquired for the future. The final session is also an opportunity to encourage the mentee to become a mentor to another mentee when appropriate.

For checklists to guide the first, follow-up and final sessions, *see* Appendix K, pp.240–1.

A framework for goal-directed interaction – GROW

A way of structuring goal-directed interaction that is relatively informal uses a sequence of enquiry described as GROW. GROW is an acronym; G is goal, R is reality – where the mentee is at now relative to their goal, O is obstacles and options for progress, and W is the way forward (Whitmore, 2009).

To use GROW as the basis of goal-directed interaction in mentoring, the mentor takes the mentee through each enquiry about the result they are seeking, their current situation, foreseeable obstacles to progress as well as options for making progress, and the mentee's decisions about the way forward.

GROW is useful because it transforms goal setting and problem solving into manageable steps. The obstacles and options (O) part of the discussion is an opportunity to introduce the topic of motivation when the mentee feels overwhelmed by the challenge of goal setting and achievement. GROW can be worked into a casual conversation to add some structure without the interaction becoming stilted.

The first goal-directed interaction session structured using GROW, begins with inviting the mentee to choose the goal they wish to work on. Next, explore the mentee's present situation relative to their goal. Consider obstacles and options for the way forward, and seek a decision from the mentee about how they will proceed. A first session structured with GROW is illustrated in Figure 16.

G oal   Desired result

⬇

R eality   Situation now

⬇

O bstacles & Options   Barriers & enablers

⬇

W ay forward   Action plan

⬇

Next session

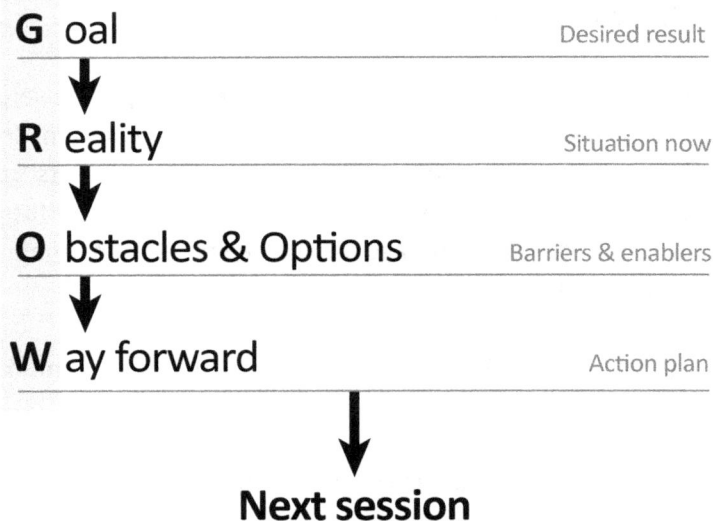

Figure 16. Structuring goal-directed interaction using GROW

A follow-up session structured using GROW, starts with exploring what the mentee did with their plan for the way forward (W), from the previous session. Did they follow through with the plan? What was the outcome? From there, return to the GROW sequence at the appropriate stage, for example by starting with a new goal (G) if the original goal was achieved, or reviewing the options and obstacles (O) related to the pursuing the original goal if the way forward (W) did not yield the desired result.

When to use goal-directed interaction

This tool is for **all** sessions.

In intentional mentoring, every session has at least one kind of goal, either to do with the developmental work or the relational work of mentoring. In the empathic attachment and felt separation stages, relational work is emphasised and goals are likely to relate to the partnership of the mentor and the mentee. In the active involvement stage, developmental work is emphasised and goals are likely to relate to the mentee's development.

Pitfalls to avoid

- Being excessively goal-directed at the expense of allowing the natural development of the partnership
- Being overly focussed on plans and goals and not noticing emerging opportunities
- Encouraging relentless pursuit of goals
- Intense and prolonged developmental work; pushing for more development too soon without recognising the mentee's achievements and need for rest
- Offering mentoring activities that are too uncomfortable or unfamiliar to the mentee, or unlikely to lead to development
- Not reviewing the mentee's aspirational state of development from time to time

Case study

To find out how Sam used this tool with Mikey during a mentoring session, turn to:

- Conversation – Partnership set-up, *see* pp.140–3
- Conversation – Learning knowledge, *see* pp.144–7
- Conversation – Learning a skill, *see* pp.148–51
- Conversation – Improving performance of an essential task, *see* pp.169–71

8. Curriculum and performance standards (Tool #4)

Case study: Being in the same specialty as Mikey meant that Sam was familiar with the curriculum and performance standards relevant to Mikey's clinical practice and training. He referred to the college curriculum as well as other familiar guidelines in order to help Mikey prepare for his exams, and made reference to the training requirements as he encouraged Mikey to continue on in his research projects.

About the tool

Performance standards are resources that describe work to be performed by the doctor, expectations of performance held by health services, the medical community and patients, and indicators of performance. In this category we include all documents that may be used as benchmarks for performance including laws, by-laws, codes of conduct, key performance indicators from job descriptions, outcome statements, patient outcome measures, error and complication rates, throughput indicators and checklists. An example is the Australian Medical Council's Intern Outcome Statements, describing outcomes to be achieved by the intern within particular domains of the intern role (AMC, 2014).

Curriculum standards are resources that describe what the doctor should know and be able to do at certain levels of seniority. This category includes lists of competencies, and lists of competencies assembled as curriculum frameworks, for example, the Australian Curriculum Framework for Junior Doctors (Confederation of Postgraduate Medical Education Councils, 2012).

What it adds to the toolkit

Curriculum and performance standards add a **focusing tool** to your toolkit. With curriculum and performance standards, the mentor and mentee can identify competency and performance requirements relevant to the mentee's cohort of doctors and use them as starting points for goal setting.

How to use the tool

Identify the curriculum and performance standards most relevant to the mentee

Some performance standards apply to all doctors (e.g. codes of conduct) and some apply to specific groups of doctors (e.g. key performance indicators from job descriptions). Curriculum standards often apply to specific groups of doctors (e.g. junior doctors). As curriculum and performance standards may be updated periodically, check for updates to ensure that your conversations with mentees are covering the most appropriate and current content. Sources of information about curriculum and performance standards include regulatory authorities, colleges and medical education units.

Be guided by curriculum and performance standards as a starting point for goal-directed interaction

As intentional mentoring offers the mentee individually-relevant assistance, generic curriculum and performance standards are treated simply as a starting point for identifying areas for the mentee to prioritise during mentoring.

Before focussing on the mentee's preparation for future roles, give priority to the mentee's performance in their current role. If the mentee does not demonstrate acceptable performance in their current role, they are unlikely to progress into senior roles.

Among managers and supervisors of doctors are diverse expectations for how the doctor role is performed. The mentee should seek to understand the expectations of each manager and supervisor in addition to formal performance standards applicable to their role.

When to use curriculum and performance standards

This tool is for **some** sessions.

During mentoring, an awareness of curriculum and performance standards relevant to the mentee's clinical practice and training provides ideas about areas to target in developmental work. Curriculum and performance standards are particularly useful at the start of mentoring when initial mentoring goals are being set.

Pitfalls to avoid

- Facilitating goal setting based only on generic curriculum and performance standards without considering the mentee's individual needs or interests
- Ignoring local or setting-specific performance standards
- Overwhelming the mentee with too many tasks associated with the curriculum and performance standards, in a short space of time

Case study

To find out how Sam used this tool with Mikey during a mentoring session, turn to:

- Conversation – Partnership set-up, *see* pp.140–3
- Conversation – Learning knowledge, *see* pp.144–7

9. Brief Intervention (Tool #5)

Case study: During mentoring, Sam helped Mikey to gain insight, improve his clinical reasoning skills, pay attention to work-life balance, and much more. Using brief interventions between scheduled mentoring conversations, Sam made the most of short amounts of time available and assisted Mikey to achieve specific results, quickly and effectively.

About the tool

A brief intervention is a short episode of facilitation that is designed to foster desired change. As a form of purposeful communication (Tool #1), the elements of a brief intervention are listening, questioning and informing. Because a brief intervention can be administered in a short space of time, it is ideal for opportunistic change efforts.

What it adds to the toolkit

Brief intervention adds an **accelerating tool** to your toolkit. Using brief intervention, a mentor can help the mentee make progress more quickly than would otherwise be possible in the time available. The mentor can also use brief intervention to assist the mentee to overcome a particular obstacle that is hindering their progress in goal achievement.

The three dimensions of development, knowing, doing and being, are targets of brief intervention. Mentors can draw from a range of theories and frameworks to facilitate specific outcomes, and also test and develop theories for what works, why, and for whom in mentoring. An example of a brief intervention is facilitating learning of knowledge, using Peyton's Set, Dialogue and Closure sequence. This involves planning and delivering teaching based on a triad of concepts: set (setting clear learning outcomes, and ensuring they are relevant, pitched at the right level, and achievable in the time available), dialogue (delivering content in ways that keep the mentee engaged) and closure (summarising take home messages and linking new learning to future self-directed learning or teaching) (Lake & Ryan, 2004). For more examples of brief interventions, loosely categorised as interventions for knowing, doing and being, *see* Appendix I, pp.225–7. In Chapter 16, p.139 a number of brief interventions will be illustrated with the help of our case study mentor and mentee duo Sam and Mikey.

How to use the tool

Decide whether a brief intervention is warranted

Not every moment is the right moment to introduce a brief intervention, even if you would like to see the mentee accelerate their progress. In mentoring and other developmental work, strain has utility as a resource for development. To offer a brief intervention too hastily may deny the mentee the opportunity to be rewarded with a breakthrough from their own efforts. Allow the mentee to try and figure out solutions or ways forward for themselves first. You can use questioning to aid this process. If the mentee is stuck and unable to progress, and you believe they will remain this way without assistance, introduce a brief intervention.

At times, an extended intervention or an intervention delivered progressively may be warranted, for example, when facilitating learning and performance of clinical reasoning, and teaching the many associated concepts and principles. Covering the concepts and principles thoroughly takes time. A starting point is identifying and focussing on one concept or principle that is deficient in the mentee's clinical reasoning and working progressively from there.

Before proceeding with a brief intervention, review your motives. The purpose of brief intervention is not to solve frustration with recalcitrant or unmotivated mentees! If frustration (or other uncomfortable emotion) associated with a lack of progress by the mentee is the driving factor, reconsider brief intervention, and make time for an accountability discussion instead.

Offer the brief intervention with a clear rationale

The effectiveness of a brief intervention depends on the mentee's level of engagement and participation in the process. How does the brief intervention relate to the goals of the mentee? What is the result you anticipate from the brief intervention? Explaining what you would like to offer, and why (the expected result), increases engagement. Any brief intervention that you offer should have clear relevance to the mentee's goals and aspirational state of development, or the interventions will appear random rather than opportunistic.

Notice the mentee's responses

As you deliver the brief intervention, pay attention to how the mentee is responding. Is the mentee engaged in the process? Does the intervention appear to make sense and have relevance to them? Is the intervention producing the intended results? Does the mentee seem to be coping with the pace of the intervention? Adjust the delivery of the intervention for maximum relevance to the mentee.

When to use brief intervention

This tool is for **some** sessions.

Intentional mentoring takes time, and brief intervention is not a substitute for making sufficient time for mentoring on a regular basis. However, the reality is that mentoring will often happen opportunistically. Brief intervention can be particularly useful at these times. It should be used in moderation because it has an opportunity cost for the mentee, the opportunity to struggle and figure out a solution for themselves. In general, if the mentee is achieving the required performance standards, is satisfied with their efforts, and has sufficient information and awareness of their choices, brief intervention is not required.

Brief interventions are also able to be used outside of a formal mentoring partnership. Developmental opportunities arise on a daily basis in the clinical environment, and a brief intervention can be a useful way to capture those opportunities with your junior medical colleagues if they are receptive and you have adequate rapport.

Pitfalls to avoid

- Delivering a brief intervention when it is unwelcome or of no interest to the mentee
- Presuming the mentee agrees to the intervention
- Administering a brief intervention that breaches the agreed scope of mentoring
- Trying to force results too soon
- Applying a brief intervention in a formulaic way, or dispensing the same intervention to all mentees irrespective of individual needs
- Pitching an intervention above the mentee's level
- Offering a brief intervention when a lengthier or more involved approach is required

Case study

To find out how Sam used this tool with Mikey during a mentoring session, turn to:

- Conversation – Learning clinical reasoning skills, *see* pp.151–5
- Conversation – Insight, *see* pp.155–9

10. Resilience work (Tool #6)

Case study: Mikey's patient died unexpectedly, and in the aftermath Sam became aware that Mikey was struggling. Sam met with Mikey to have a conversation about what Mikey was experiencing and how he was coping. Sam mentioned professional counselling as a resource, and offered guidance based on his own experience.

About the tool

Before defining resilience work we briefly examine the concept of resilience, adopting Epstein and Krasner's (2013) definition which highlights the connection between resilience and stress.

> "Resilience is the ability of an individual to respond to stress in a healthy, adaptive way such that personal goals are achieved at minimal psychological and physical cost; resilient individuals not only "bounce back" rapidly after challenges but also grow stronger in the process." (p. 301)

A note on terminology in this chapter: *Stress* (or stress response) is the cascade of physical and biochemical reactions to a perceived threat to homeostasis. It is helpful for survival when it is triggered and resolved, but it is harmful when it is triggered chronically and without resolution. A *stressor* (also known as stress stimulus), is the perceived threat (Maté, 2003). Our use of the term *stress management* refers to the mentee's management of both stress and stressors.

Resilience work is a type of goal-directed interaction (Tool #3) that focuses on assisting the mentee to acquire sustained resilience. It has three components: stress management work, energy management work, and self-preservation work. Energy is the "capacity to carry out an action" (Siegel, 2010, p. 52) and is the fuel for effective stress management, so energy management is part of resilience work. For the intense giving of oneself that medical practice requires, the preserving of oneself is a prerequisite, and this too is a focus of resilience work.

What it adds to the toolkit

Resilience work adds a **fortifying tool** to your toolkit. It provides ways of engaging with the mentee in relation to their strategies for stress and energy management and self-preservation. It encourages the mentee to develop self-awareness and healthy coping strategies. It teaches the mentee resilient behaviours to help them "shift the focus from pathological stress to successful adaptation" (Jensen, Trollope-Kumar, Waters & Everson, 2008, p.727) and become a resilient doctor.

Building on Epstein and Krasner's definition of individual resilience, we propose that a resilient doctor is one who:

- engages with stressors in a healthy way
- actively notices and resolves their stress responses
- finds ways to achieve goals without undue psychological and physical cost
- grows stronger through challenges
- has an energy source for action and endurance
- expends energy wisely and renews their energy reserves
- attends to self-preservation including preserving their health, values, morale and sense of self as a whole person.

The mentee's efforts to acquire sustained resilience are not just for their benefit, but also for the benefit of patients.

> "Patients want physicians who are attentive, rested, present, and caring. They want physicians with the resilience to handle stress that may be the result of their own and other patients' devastating illnesses and complex problems. They want physicians who can recognize potential errors before they happen, slow down when they should, seek advice when they are overwhelmed, and respond mindfully rather than react reflexively to complex and challenging situations. They want physicians who are sufficiently connected to other physicians to draw support, advice, information, and wisdom."
> (Epstein & Krasner, 2013, p.303)

With resilience, doctors increase the quality of care they provide to patients, and reduce errors, burnout and attrition from the medical workforce (Epstein & Krasner, 2013). Effective resilience work contributes to these results.

How to use the tool

Work on stress management

By working with the mentee on stress management, your aim is to assist the mentee to engage with stressors and manage stress in healthy, effective ways. The mentee's ability to notice stress (self-monitor), and restore calm and ease (self-regulate) without generating new stress and stressors, are indicators of healthy, effective stress management.

The work begins with assisting the mentee to become familiar with their own unique stressors. Stressors may be external stressors, stimuli external to the mentee, such as:

- demands and expectations of others, assigned responsibilities
- long hours, heavy workloads, deadlines
- behaviour of colleagues, relationship difficulties, conflict, bullying
- performance assessment, feedback delivered poorly
- competition for scarce training places, barriers to goal achievement, lack of resources.

Stressors may also be internal stressors, stimuli within the mentee, for example:

- perfectionism, self-criticism, feelings of inadequacy, worry, indecision
- inability to say no, taking on too many responsibilities, commitments, habits of disorganisation
- physical tension, health conditions, injuries, pain, hunger.

In the research literature, three factors identified as universally leading to stress are uncertainty, lack of information and loss of control (Maté, 2003), and all are realities of medical practice.

What are the mentee's responses to stressors – in what ways do they experience stress? The relationship between stress stimulus and response is unique to the individual. What does the mentee do to restore calm and ease? Of the mentee's stress management strategies, some will be more helpful than others in restoring calm and ease without generating new stressors and stress. Excessive alcohol consumption is an example of a strategy that may produce calm and ease, but also produce new stressors such as health, relationship, performance and financial problems. Assist the mentee to identify their most adaptive and values-consistent strategies for stress management, and decide a plan for implementing and reviewing the effectiveness of their strategies.

Work on energy management

By working with the mentee on energy management, your aim is to assist the mentee with managing their energy so that they have endurance and the capacity to encounter stressors and carry out action for as long as action is needed. Anticipating energy requirements relative to energy reserves, having ways to renew energy and build an energy reserve, and offsetting energy drains (experiences that have a de-energising effect) with energy gains (experiences that have an energising effect) are key indicators of effective energy management.

Like stress management, energy management relies on awareness combined with effective action. The dimensions of development, knowing, doing and being, are useful in guiding the mentee's efforts to manage their energy effectively. Ideally, the mentee actively translates gains in one dimension to the other dimensions. For example, the mentee:

- notices symptoms of fatigue due to working excessive hours on an ongoing basis and makes a conscious decision to make time for rest and sleep (knowing)
- incorporates sufficient rest and sleep into their schedule (doing)
- decides that resilience is a value that they will uphold as an ongoing direction, and chooses to be a doctor who balances self-care and other-care (being).

Work on self-preservation

Being a helping professional requires the "intense giving of oneself to enhance the lives of others" (Skovholt & Trotter-Mathison, 2016, p. xvii). By working with the mentee on self-preservation, your aim is to assist the mentee with their capacity for giving oneself without losing oneself. Preserving health, values, morale and a sense of self as a whole person are indicators of self-preservation.

Protect The Caring Self

Skovholt and Trotter-Mathison (2016) quote Kierkegaard's words "haemorrhaging of the Caring Self" in describing how the Caring Self, an aspect of one's self as a helper, can be affected by work in the helping professions (p.101). They note five spears that can stab at the helping professional's Caring Self: burnout, compassion fatigue, vicarious trauma, ambiguous endings and professional uncertainty. *The Resilient Practitioner* (Skovholt & Trotter-Mathison, 2016) and *Help for the Helper* (Rothschild, 2006) are resources containing a wealth of information relevant to both mentors and mentees who wish to learn more about these experiences and how to manage and prevent them.

Prevent demoralization and assist with remoralization

Demoralization, in its most basic form, is a loss of morale due to a feeling of subjective incompetence (Gabel, 2013). Demoralization has five main dimensions: a loss of meaning, dysphoria, disheartenment, helplessness and a sense of failure. Most, if not all doctors have experienced demoralization at some point in their career. Indeed, for some doctors it seems to sit just under the surface. For many, it is a confirmation of imposter syndrome, a false belief that one has somehow fluked their way through their training thus far, and live in fear of being found out. Demoralization can occur when someone has this insecurity affirmed.

Demoralization is also associated with morals and values; demoralization can occur when there are severe threats to an individual's core values or personal goals (Gabel, 2011). It will come as no surprise to most readers that these events are common in the daily lives of junior doctors.

Demoralization can lead to one of two clusters of detrimental thoughts and behaviours. The first is the cluster of depression, angst and burnout, which can lead to career change and major mental illness. The second is the cluster of cynicism, emotional exhaustion and depersonalisation (Leiter, Frank & Matheson, 2009). This cluster is often seen in the jaded senior doctor, who may inadvertently contribute to a demoralising culture for junior medical colleagues.

Several methods have been suggested to prevent demoralization and assist with remoralization, including continuing professional development programs, mindfulness and Balint groups (Gabel, 2013). Mentoring may also prevent demoralization, both in the mentor and in the mentee. In mentoring, guided well-being questions are invaluable in assisting the mentee to identify demoralization as an issue. Offering encouragement and perspective are ways that a mentor can help a mentee to avoid demoralization, while the enthusiasm and idealism of the mentee can help the mentor to avoid cynicism.

Use Purposeful communication (Tool #1), Partnership (Tool #2), Goal-directed interaction (Tool #3) and Confidentiality (Tool #8)

Four other tools from the intentional mentor's toolkit are particularly important in resilience work. In this section we highlight the relevance of aspects of these tools.

Use purposeful communication (Tool #1)

Understand the mentee's baseline functioning – Understanding the mentee's baseline functioning provides a reference point for recognising changes to the mentee's behaviours, cognitions and emotions over the course of mentoring. It also allows you to recognise the mentee's needs for support, and gauge effectiveness of mentoring activities and interventions. Understanding the mentee's baseline functioning involves forming an impression of the types of behaviours, cognitions and emotions that are typical for the mentee under normal circumstances. This information can be gathered naturally through conversations and interactions over time. The elements of purposeful communication, listening, questioning and informing, are important here.

Listen, question and inform – In resilience work, listening, questioning and informing have a focus on fostering resilience, for example:
- Listening – listening to allow the mentee to express themselves and feel heard and understood; paying attention to cues about the mentee's functioning relative to their baseline functioning
- Questioning – asking the mentee to imagine themselves at their most resilient and to describe how they would be functioning; checking with the mentee your impressions and assumptions about the mentee's well-being
- Informing – using encouraging and validating words; giving permission for the mentee to talk about themselves and their feelings; reminding the mentee about what to look out for as symptoms of overwhelm, burnout and other experiences of 'dis-ease'

Support, challenge and facilitate – Supporting, challenging and facilitating are all relevant to resilience work, for example:
- Supporting – reassuring the mentee that they are not alone with their challenges; validating what the mentee is experiencing
- Challenging – encouraging the mentee to set limits and learn to say no at times; encouraging the mentee to step out of the role of helper at times and accept help; encouraging the mentee to do more of what makes them stronger as a whole person
- Facilitating – facilitating the mentee's awareness, monitoring and regulation of their stress responses and energy levels

Use partnership (Tool #2)

Take care with boundaries – Ideally, the mentee will proactively establish and maintain a support network including friends, family, colleagues and a general practitioner. Know where your mentor role begins and ends within the mentee's support network, and how your role fits with the roles of other support people. The mentor role is to do relational and developmental work with the mentee and add structure to mentoring, so that the mentee develops as a doctor in practice. It is not advisable to be the primary support person for a mentee having an exaggerated grief reaction or suffering from mental illness that warrants healthcare from a mental health professional. In these circumstances, your contribution can be as a facilitator to ensure that the mentee is receiving the healthcare they require.

Ensure access to appropriate healthcare – Doctors have a greater rate of very high levels of psychological distress, than other groups of professionals (*beyondblue*, 2013). If you believe that the mentee is experiencing very high levels of psychological distress, direct communication is vital. Ask the mentee what they are experiencing and ensure they have access to appropriate healthcare.

Use goal-directed interaction (Tool #3)

Tailor the work to the individual mentee – An effective mentoring partnership functions as a safe space for the mentee to explore resilience and strategies for building and sustaining resilience. The work should be tailored to the individual mentee because stressors, stress responses, coping mechanisms and resources are unique to the mentee.

Assist the mentee to develop a resilience repertoire – Jensen et al. (2008) identify four dynamic elements associated with resilience in family physicians: attitudes and perspectives, balance and prioritisation, practice management and supportive relations. These elements may be used as themes to explore in your resilience work with the mentee, and for setting resilience goals. Ideally, resilience work will result in the mentee building an individually-relevant 'resilience repertoire', a repertoire of knowing (a dynamic knowledge and skills base), doing (a set of performance behaviours) and being (awareness and practise of values) related to resilience. An example of a resilience repertoire is shown in Figure 17. A comprehensive aspirational state of development contains a resilience repertoire.

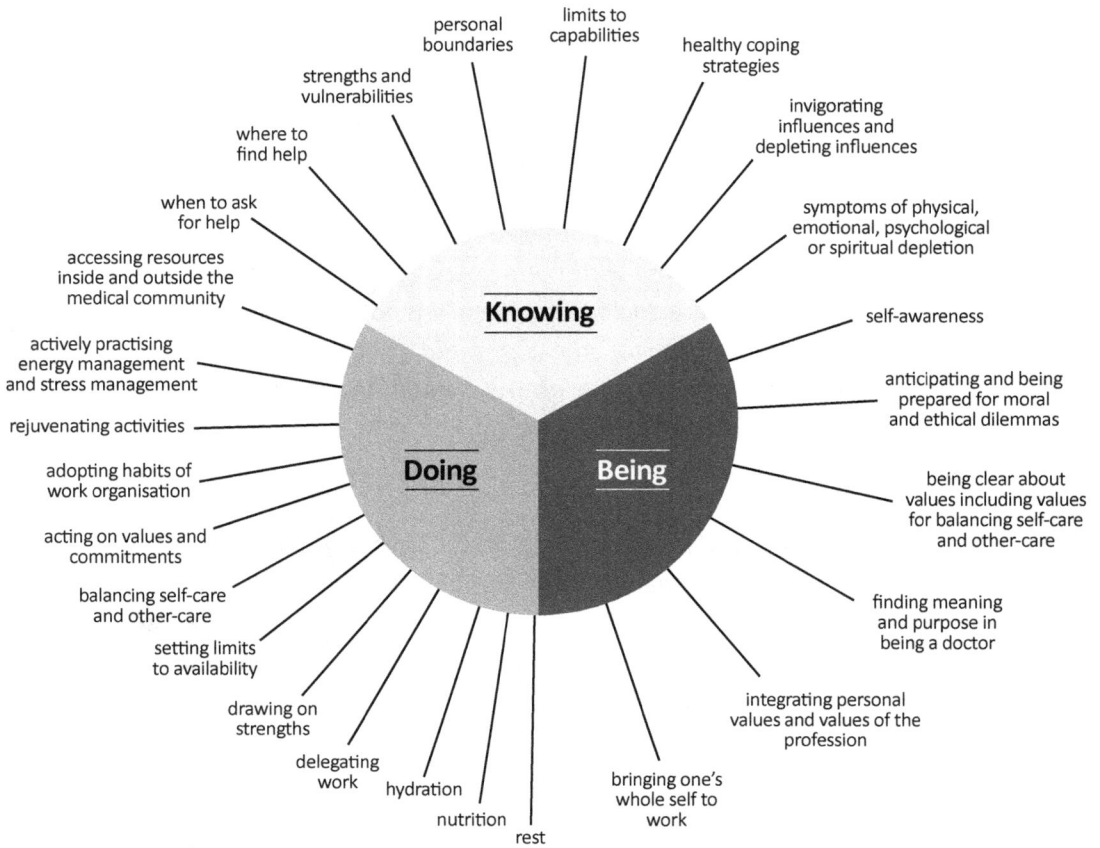

Figure 17. A resilience repertoire

Draw from evidence-based methods – The practice of mindfulness is increasingly being recognised as an effective contributor to resilience. Mindfulness is a type of awareness that involves paying attention to the present moment with an attitude of openness, receptivity and curiosity. Mindfulness combined with values-focused action is a powerful approach to well-being, and is used in Acceptance and Commitment Therapy (Hayes & Smith, 2005). The approach can also be used in mentoring to assist the mentee to manage their thoughts and feelings effectively, rise above uncomfortable thoughts and feelings, and be free to pursue what matters most.

For a brief summary of prominent evidence-based approaches to fostering resilience and quality of life, *see* Appendix J, p.229. While these approaches are commonly used as frameworks for counselling and coaching, they may also be sources of ideas for resilience work in mentoring for those readers wishing to acquire advanced skills.

Use confidentiality (Tool #8)

Recognise vulnerability, and follow up – The mentee's disclosure of personal issues related to resilience and well-being is an act of trust that should not be taken lightly. The mentee may experience vulnerability in making disclosures, and is likely to regret making disclosures if they do not receive reassurance of the mentor's care and concern. When you follow up with the mentee you reassure them that they are not alone with what they are facing, and you have the opportunity to inform the mentee of resources available to them that are relevant to their needs.

Seek advice if necessary – Mandatory reporting requirements prevail in the event that the mentee is affected by a health issue that impairs practice and places the public at risk of harm (AHPRA, 2016). In this situation, seek immediate advice from the appropriate regulatory agency.

A framework for resilience work – The Eye of the Storm Model of Practitioner Resiliency

The Eye of the Storm Model of Practitioner Resiliency (Skovholt & Trotter-Mathison, 2016) offers an approach to sustaining resilience over the long term, and is for all people in helping-caring, relationship-intense professions, including the medical profession, where there is giving of oneself to enhance the lives of others. The Eye of the Storm Model of Practitioner Resiliency features in *The Resilient Practitioner* (Skovholt & Trotter-Mathison, 2016). The model has special significance to *The Intentional Mentor in Medicine*; a mainstay of the model, like this book, is the Cycle of Caring.

The eye of the storm is a metaphor for the quiet space where the patient and doctor work together in the helping relationship. The doctor sits on a three-legged stool. Around the doctor, the storm of the patient's suffering swirls. While the doctor supports the patient, the three legs of the stool support the doctor. The three-legged stool is a metaphor for three keys to practitioner resilience, based upon pursuit of:

1. a high vitality index; tapping into sources of vitality (energy, hope and optimism) and actively reducing sources of personal and professional stress
2. expertise in the Cycle of Caring applied to medical practice (a four-phase cycle including re-creation); using success of the helping process as a performance indicator, and combining generosity in giving with deep self-care for the long-term, to be able to continue to give

3. the intense will to learn and grow (one especially powerful source of vitality); committing to learning and developing, stretching oneself, being open to feedback, and using defining moments to grow as a doctor, resulting in increased competency, sense of accomplishment and energy.

In your mentor role, The Eye of the Storm Model of Practitioner Resiliency can help you to focus the mentee's attention on these three keys to sustaining resilience.

When to use resilience work

This tool is for **all** sessions.

Resilience work belongs in all mentoring encounters. It starts with asking the mentee "How are you?" as a meaningful and important question about how they are doing, and how they are coping with the demands of work, not just as part of a greeting. It involves taking the time to listen carefully to the mentee's answer, and to explore their answer if any part of the response is concerning.

Pitfalls to avoid

- Trying to fulfil needs of the mentee that fall outside the scope of mentoring
- Pathologising feelings that are normal reactions to difficult situations
- Not following up with the mentee about well-being issues disclosed
- Being unavailable to the mentee at the agreed times
- Displaying discomfort when the mentee expresses distress
- Not listening actively to the mentee

Case study

To find out how Sam used this tool with Mikey during a mentoring session, turn to:

- Conversation – Well-being, *see* pp.159–61
- Conversation – Accountability, *see* pp.162–5
- Conversation – Work-life balance, *see* pp.172–3
- Conversation – Understanding and addressing performance problems that are complex, *see* pp.166–9

11. Career guidance (Tool #7)

Case study: During their initial discussion, Sam and Mikey talked about what Mikey wanted his career to look like. Was he interested in becoming a clinician, a researcher or an academic? Perhaps all three, or none at all? The goals that were set were in line with Mikey's desire to become a clinician, but both Sam and Mikey were cognisant that Mikey's exposure to other aspects of medicine were limited. Hence, there was deliberate effort to expose Mikey to areas including research, to see if Mikey found them appealing. Sam was keen to offer Mikey guidance on how to advance his career path, and was also happy to assist in practical ways, such as being his referee and supervising a research project.

About the tool

Career guidance is goal-directed interaction (Tool #3) that relates specifically to career. Career guidance assists the mentee to identify and acquire knowledge and skills, performance behaviours, and values that are helpful for navigating the training pathways towards a particular type of career in medicine.

What it adds to the toolkit

Career guidance adds a **navigating tool** to your toolkit. Career guidance as a tool for development is useful for guiding the mentee to resources, opportunities and pathways for career advancement. Career guidance is also useful for assisting the mentee to make decisions related to career, such as their desired lifestyle, the location of the career, and the timeframe for pursuing the career, and to prepare for the many moments of transition they will experience along the way during their developmental journey.

How to use the tool

Identify the mentee's vision of their place in the profession

If you were to survey a group of mentees, you would likely find a variety of states of awareness about career path preferences. Some mentees have well-formed ideas from medical school or earlier years, and others remain uncertain about the direction they want to take after several years of working. Some mentees have it down to a couple of different options. Not only is it good to work out what the mentee's place on that spectrum of awareness is, but also the reasons behind their choice/s. Reasons for choosing a specialty are many and varied, but usually include a combination of one or more of the following:

- Passion and enjoyment – how much they like the 'fun' parts of the job
- Tolerability – how well they are able to tolerate the mundane or unpleasant parts of the job
- Earning potential
- Lifestyle and family considerations
- Entry requirements to the training program
- Time and energy commitment of the training program
- External influences (e.g. family expectations, role models)
- Altruism – a sense of responsibility to meet the needs of a community

Each of these reasons will have different levels of importance for different doctors. It can be worthwhile helping the mentee identify which is most important to them now, what is likely to be important to them in the future, and where conflicts might arise.

Some will want to, and have, the ability to become world experts in a field. Passion is likely to top the list for them. Others may want a career that affords them lots of time with family, friends and other activities. Whilst these two goals are not mutually exclusive, they may be practically exclusive depending on the individual's circumstances, so appropriate counselling may be needed. It is important to address any incongruence in goals.

Encourage the mentee to find a direction that is consistent with their interests, strengths and what matters most to them. Finding something that they are able to commit to wholeheartedly and have no doubts about, will make their journey easier.

It is worth remembering that in general, training is not like consultant practice. Most hospital-based training happens in tertiary centres where the trainers are full-time public consultants, occasionally with research interests. In this environment trainees may not be cognisant of the other options within the field of medicine, such as private practice, corporate work, education or full-time research/academia.

Connect the mentee to current and reliable resources

Supporting the mentee's access to resources means connecting them to people and materials that will help them make progress that is relevant to their preferred career path. This is particularly important if the mentee is interested in pursuing a field different to the mentor's field. Asking a colleague in the field of interest for help will assist you to counsel the mentee appropriately.

Wilson and Feyer (2015) recommend that career planning across the medical education continuum be aligned with societal health and medical workforce needs, stating:

> "...Valid career aspirations of students and graduates are framed by a good understanding of future workforce needs and expectations of training as well as appraisal of their own skills. Neither the individual nor the system benefits from graduates collectively aspiring to a narrow range of career choices when community needs are in fact much broader." (p. 24)

Explore with the mentee:

- a broad range of career paths
- projected workforce needs and expected future demands for specialists
- entry requirements and success rates for entry into vocational training programs
- long-term career opportunities, employment prospects and whether specialties are under or over-subscribed
- work opportunities with regards to their aspirational state of development (e.g. academia, research, public clinical work, private clinical work, part-time, full-time, administration).

Work collaboratively towards goal achievement

After goals are decided, assist the mentee to achieve their goals. *See* Chapter 7, pp.85–8 for guidelines on facilitating goal achievement.

When to use career guidance

This tool is for **some** sessions.

Because the developmental journey of a doctor is a series of transitions, with performance, career advancement and resilience interactive elements of the journey, career decisions should be a regular part of the work that you do with the mentee.

Pitfalls to avoid

- Not exploring the mentee's reasons for choosing a career path
- Limiting the discussion of training options to local options instead of looking further afield and using creativity to solve issues of access
- Persuading the mentee to follow the career path of the mentor
- Neglecting long term consideration of life beyond training
- Failing to understand and factor in the mentee's personal and social circumstances (e.g. family commitments and requirements to relocate) when exploring career options
- Forgetting to discuss non-clinical specialties (e.g. administration, pathology)

Case study

To find out how Sam used this tool with Mikey during a mentoring session, turn to:

- Conversation – Partnership set-up, *see* pp.140–3
- Conversation – Work-life balance, *see* pp.172–3

12. Confidentiality (Tool #8)

Case study: During mentoring, Sam received personal and sensitive information from Mikey, particularly around the time when Mikey was dealing with the possible mental illness of a colleague that was affecting the colleague's work performance. Sam was aware at all times of his responsibilities in regards to confidentiality. Sam shared some of his own personal information with Mikey to show empathy and help Mikey through a difficult situation. This was a considered decision by Sam, and he shared the information, trusting in their confidentiality agreement.

About the tool

Confidentiality is the protection of confidential information. It is a universal expectation when dealing with personal and sensitive information in the workplace. It is also essential for building trust, a mainstay of partnership. Mentors should make themselves familiar with the different local, state and federal laws and policies that govern privacy and confidentiality in their jurisdiction.

What it adds to the toolkit

Confidentiality adds a **safety tool** to your toolkit. In mentoring, confiding of personal and sensitive information is commonplace, and confidentiality helps the mentor and the mentee to feel safe in making disclosures and participating in activities that are conducive to the mentee's development. Confidentiality also provides safety from a legal perspective. The mentor's and mentee's compliance with privacy and confidentiality requirements prevents legal problems associated with improper management of personal and sensitive information.

How to use the tool

Understand laws relevant to your mentoring practice

In Australia, a number of privacy laws apply to the management of personal and sensitive information within health and other services, relating to the collection, use, disclosure and storage of information. The Office of the Australian Information Commissioner website provides resources and guidance (https://www.oaic.gov.au). In general, the permitted collection, use, disclosure and storage of information, is the collection, use, disclosure and storage specified at the time of collection.

Give the mentee an explanation of how your information management practices are law-abiding

During the partnership set-up phase, discuss expectations in regards to confidentiality and limits to confidentiality. This should include your intentions for lawful collection, use, disclosure and storage of information about the mentee. As mentoring involves sharing of personal and sensitive information, confidentiality should be a two-way agreement; you will protect the mentee's confidential information and they will do likewise.

Discuss and decide whether to keep any records of mentoring

Records of mentoring may be kept by the mentor and or the mentee, such as a log of meeting dates, discussion topics and progress. If you are working with a number of mentees it may be difficult to keep track of what each mentee is up to or gather evaluation data without keeping any records. If you decide to keep records of mentoring, you are responsible for storing the records securely.

Keep your promises to the mentee to protect their privacy

After promising the mentee that you will treat their information confidentially, your responsibility is to uphold your commitment. Discuss with the mentee any requests you receive to release information about them, and obtain their agreement in writing prior to the release of information.

Notifiable conduct presents a challenging information management situation in mentoring. In Australia, notifiable conduct by registered health practitioners is defined by the Australian Health Practitioner Regulation Agency (AHPRA) as:

- practising while intoxicated by alcohol or drugs
- sexual misconduct in the practice of the profession
- placing the public at risk of substantial harm because of an impairment (health issue), or
- placing the public at risk because of a significant departure from accepted professional standards (AHPRA, 2016).

If you have to report the mentee for notifiable conduct, the mentoring partnership is likely to end. Although this puts you in a difficult position, it is necessary to escalate some situations to the appropriate authorities when the mentee's behaviour puts the public at risk. The mentee should be made aware from the start of the partnership that notifiable conduct is reportable.

When to use confidentiality

This tool is for **all** sessions.

Confidentiality applies throughout the mentoring partnership as an ongoing responsibility. At times, confidentiality will be an overt discussion point, for example, while negotiating the mentoring agreement and coming to an understanding of the ways you will manage personal and sensitive information, or when responding to a request from the mentee for a record of their participation in mentoring.

Pitfalls to avoid

- Sharing or releasing information about the mentee without the mentee's permission
- Storing information about the mentee in a way that is not secure
- Not discussing with the mentee what constitutes notifiable conduct, at the start of the partnership

- Not reporting notifiable conduct by the mentee, because of a significant personal affection or friendship
- Not reporting notifiable conduct by the mentee, due to a lack of knowledge of regulations about what must be reported, versus what may be kept confidential

Case study

To find out how Sam used this tool with Mikey during a mentoring session, turn to:

- Conversation – Partnership set-up, *see* pp.140–3
- Conversation – Well-being, *see* pp.159–61
- Conversation – Understanding and addressing performance problems that are complex, *see* pp.166–9

13. Evaluation (Tool #9)

Case study: Throughout mentoring, Sam continued to monitor Mikey's goal achievement and movement towards his aspirational state of development. Periodically, Sam and Mikey evaluated their mentoring process and outcomes. When Mikey failed to make progress with his research, Sam facilitated a discussion to review what had happened and what resulted, and whether a research paper remained a realistic goal. After the discussion, the plan for goal achievement was adjusted. At the conclusion of mentoring, Sam and Mikey reflected together on their contributions to the mentoring process, and the outcomes, over the course of the two-year partnership.

About the tool

Evaluation is a set of activities used to increase understanding of one or more aspects of mentoring. The essential activities of evaluation are deciding on the purpose of the evaluation, forming questions to answer, collecting data, analysing data, interpreting the results and acting on the findings.

What it adds to the toolkit

Evaluation adds a **discovery tool** to your toolkit, creating opportunities for noticing and understanding various aspects of the mentoring process and outcomes in your work with the mentee. A key concern is establishing not just whether the mentee achieved their goals and developed as a doctor, but also whether mentoring contributed to the results, and if so, how. A two-part evaluation sequence of process evaluation and outcome evaluation yields this understanding.

Both process and outcome evaluation use the same activities: deciding on the purpose of evaluation, forming questions, collecting data, analysing data, interpreting the results and acting on findings. However, process evaluation focuses on describing what happened during and around mentoring, while outcome evaluation focuses on ascertaining the results of mentoring.

Inputs, activities and outputs are three types of information that are central to process evaluation (Centers for Disease Control and Prevention (CDC), 2008; MacDonald et al., 2001). In intentional mentoring, *inputs* are the resources invested and used, such as the mentor's and mentee's time and materials. *Activities* are how the inputs are converted into actions in mentoring, for example, mentoring conversations. *Outputs* are the products of mentoring, usually described in numerical terms, including the quantity of activities. Together, inputs, activities and outputs describe the mentoring that occurred. Contextual information is also recognised and utilised in process evaluation to understand what was happening around mentoring at the time mentoring occurred. Process evaluation information is carried over to outcome evaluation, to identify the effects of the mentoring process on outcomes (results).

Figure 18 illustrates the two-part enquiry that is process and outcome evaluation. Together, the process and outcome evaluations tell the results of mentoring and the story behind the results.

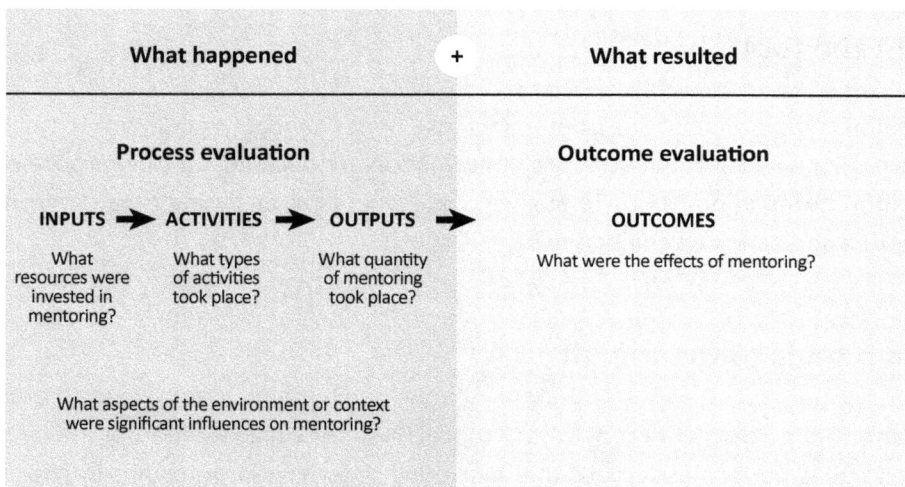

What happened	+	**What resulted**
Process evaluation		**Outcome evaluation**
INPUTS ➡ ACTIVITIES ➡ OUTPUTS ➡		OUTCOMES
What resources were invested in mentoring? What types of activities took place? What quantity of mentoring took place?		What were the effects of mentoring?
What aspects of the environment or context were significant influences on mentoring?		

Figure 18. An overview of process and outcome evaluation

How to use the tool

Plan evaluation

The sequence of process and outcome evaluation is scalable and can be applied to a brief intervention within a mentoring session, a whole mentoring session, a series of mentoring sessions, or the entire partnership and process. Evaluation should be planned in advance, including questions, sources of data (e.g. mentoring conversations and records), methods of analysis, and measures of success, to ensure the required information is gathered and processed in a timely way.

When seeking to evaluate an entire partnership and process, a common challenge is recognising a clear starting point for mentoring. Mentoring partnerships often have an incubation phase during which the mentor delivers individually-relevant support, challenge and facilitation, yet an agreement has not been reached to enter a partnership. The time of acceptance of the roles of mentor and mentee serves as a clear start point for mentoring.

Notice what happened

For a defined interval, notice what happened in and around mentoring. The most basic way to do this is to ask and answer questions related to process, for example:

- To what extent did the mentee engage in mentoring?
- Did the mentee perceive you as the mentor to be committed, accessible, responsive and engaged?
- What types and quantity of activities took place?
- What resources were invested?
- Did the mentee receive encouragement from their organisation to participate in mentoring?
- Was mentoring implemented as planned?

Notice what resulted

For a defined interval, notice what resulted from mentoring. Examples of questions to ask and answer are:

- What were the effects of mentoring on the mentee's knowledge and skills, performance, and awareness and practise of values?
- What goals did the mentee achieve as a result of mentoring?
- How did mentoring change the care that the mentee's patients received?
- Did mentoring yield the expected results?
- What effects did mentoring have, that were unexpected?

An experimental design is generally the strongest design for establishing a cause-effect relationship (Berg & Latin, 2011). In the context of mentoring, the most basic experimental design is a pre/post study which refers to those studies where measurement(s) are taken before the intervention, and then the same measurements are repeated after the intervention. This allows measurement of any changes that have occurred due to the mentoring. However, it can be difficult to attribute any observed changes solely to mentoring, in the absence of a control group.

Decide what to pay attention to as measures of success

If an aim of evaluation is to determine the success of mentoring, success requires definition. With the mentee, decide on the definition of success (e.g. what success would look and feel like to the mentee) and meaningful measures of success. This applies to both process and outcome evaluation.

Process indicators are the specific, observable measures of inputs, activities and outputs used in process evaluation. In mentoring, examples of process indicators include the number of mentoring conversations, topics of conversation, and types and quantity of mentoring activities. On its own, process evaluation information is neutral and remains purely descriptive until you establish standards to compare it with. The contents of the mentoring agreement (e.g. the agreed frequency of mentoring conversations), serve as standards.

Outcome indicators are the specific, observable measures of the effects of mentoring used in outcome evaluation. In mentoring, examples of outcome indicators include goal achievement, job offers, successful applications to vocational training programs, and improved results of assessments and tasks such as those administered by employers and training agencies, illustrated in Figure 19.

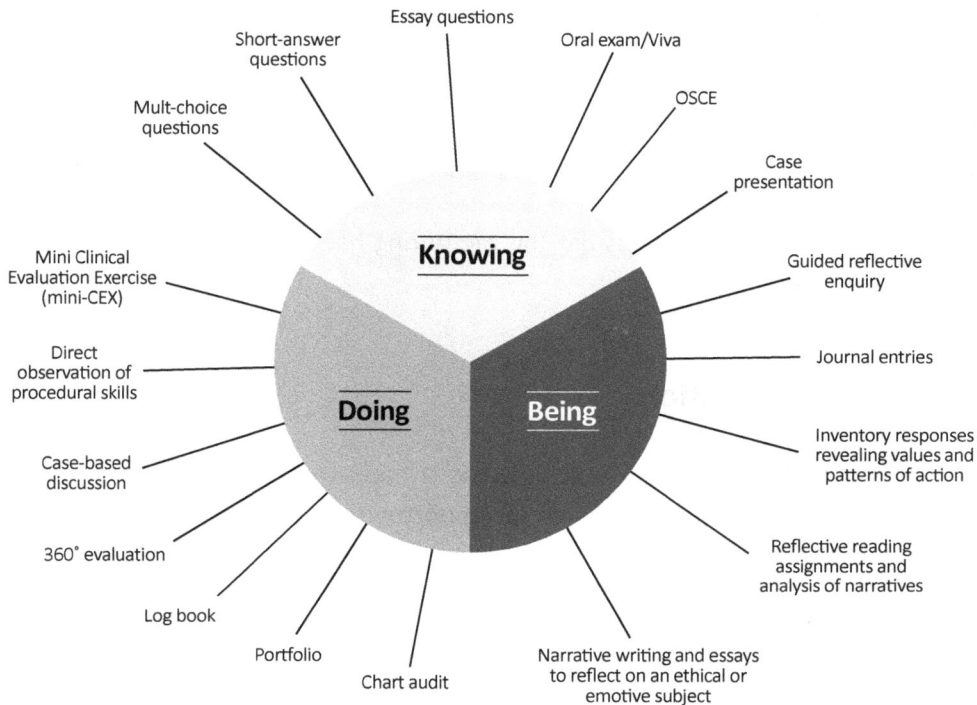

Figure 19. Assessment data sources

Use findings to improve future mentoring

Evaluation findings are useful for improving mentoring for an individual mentee, and for making decisions about future mentoring. A determined mentor and mentee in partnership try many activities until they find the ones that bring about the desired results. This involves the mentor and mentee paying attention to results, continuing to do what works, and discontinuing what does not work. Evaluation findings are also useful for generating theory about what works, why, and for whom in mentoring.

A framework for evaluation – Kirkpatrick's hierarchy

Kirkpatrick's hierarchy is a framework commonly used in medical education to conduct evaluation that incorporates process and outcome evaluation (Kirkpatrick, 1967). It has four levels of enquiry, Level 1 reaction, Level 2 learning, Level 3 behaviour and Level 4 results.

The questions you form can be based on these levels. For example,

Level 1 (Reaction) – Is the mentee satisfied with their experiences of mentoring?

Level 2 Learning) – Did the mentee increase their knowledge and skills through mentoring?

Level 3 (Behaviour) – Did the mentee apply any of the knowledge or skills they gained through mentoring?

Level 4 (Results) – What impacts did the mentoring have on patient outcomes, the organisation or the community?

When to use evaluation

This tool is for **all** sessions. By noticing what is happening in mentoring and what results are being produced, you have an opportunity to adjust what you offer to positively influence the mentoring process and outcomes. Evaluation does not have to be complicated. Even a simple question like "Was this helpful for you?" yields clues about the mentee's experience and what to adjust during future mentoring.

Pitfalls to avoid

- Considering the contributions of only the mentor or the mentee to the mentoring process
- A reductionist approach, measuring parts of mentoring too small to be meaningful
- Applying the same definition of success to each mentoring partnership
- Ignoring unintended effects of mentoring
- Limiting outcome measures to highly visible measures of success such as a successful vocational training program application
- Not acting on evaluation findings

Case study

To find out how Sam used this tool with Mikey during a mentoring session, turn to:

- Conversation – Accountability, *see* pp.162–5
- Conversation – Concluding mentoring, *see* pp.173–8

14. Reflective practice of mentoring (Tool #10)

Case study: During the course of mentoring, Sam continually reviewed his performance as a mentor to identify ways he could improve his relational and developmental work, and be an effective mentor to Mikey.

About the tool

Reflective practice of mentoring is a way of studying personal experiences of practice to acquire knowledge, insights and commitments for future practice.

What it adds to the toolkit

Reflective practice of mentoring adds a **self-monitoring tool** to your toolkit. It requires you to reflect on the developmental and relational work you do with the mentee, identify your contributions and experiences, and plan for how you will conduct yourself during future mentoring.

How to use the tool

Reflect during each encounter with the mentee

Reflection in action is reflection that takes places during activity. It allows for awareness of what is transpiring, and for adjusting the activity while it is in progress (Schon, 1987). It is particularly useful for enacting intentional mentoring principles of constructiveness and productivity, that is, relating positively and doing more of what works for the development of the mentee. If an activity is not working in service of the mentee's goal/s, reflection in action enables noticing and redesigning the activity for a better result.

Reflect after each encounter with the mentee

Reflection on action is the reflection that takes place after the activity to discover how thoughts and actions led to results (Schon, 1987). If you have time after an interaction with the mentee, even if it is only for a minute or two, consider how the interaction went. What took place during the interaction? What knowledge, skills and tools did you apply? What decisions and choices did you make in structuring the interaction, and why?

As you reflect, turn your attention to yourself and your reactions to the interaction. What was the significance of the interaction to you? If the interaction elicited difficult emotions, consider how you will manage the emotions and issues that surfaced, in a way that is not detrimental to the mentee.

Evaluate your contribution to mentoring

Reflective practice and evaluation share some common ground, as they both involve noticing what happened and what resulted in mentoring. However, reflective practice places the focus on understanding your contributions to the process and outcomes. Questions that are relevant include: What did you contribute to the relational and developmental work of the interaction? Did you show CARE? Were you prepared for the interaction?

Determine actions to adjust your practice if required

If you reflect and notice that your contributions to mentoring were less than you had hoped for – or conversely, your contributions demanded more of your time and energy than you had allowed for – consider the actions you will take to adjust your future mentoring practice. You could adjust the times and locations of interactions, and or the types of activities you offer. You could also adjust your preparedness for future mentoring by acquiring new skills, such as skills in facilitating learning, or skills for assertiveness and saying no to requests for assistance if the mentee is asking for more than you are prepared to give. Consider how you might incorporate the lessons from reflection into your future mentoring practice, for example, by establishing clear boundaries at the beginning of new partnerships.

Join or form a mentoring community of practice

Chapter 2 introduced communities of practice as "groups of people who share a concern or a passion for something they do and learn how to do it better as they interact regularly" (Wenger-Trayner & Wenger-Trayner, 2015, p.1). By joining or forming a community of practice with other mentors, you have the opportunity to share experiences of mentoring, exchange ideas and resources, and learn methods and techniques that can be applied in your work with mentees. If a formal mentoring program exists at your workplace, the program coordinator may be able to connect you to an existing mentoring community of practice, or assist you to establish one in your practice setting.

Monitor the impacts of mentoring on you, and balance self-care and other-care

Mentoring can be taxing, particularly if many mentees are seeking your assistance, or if you are involved in clinical training in a number of ways (e.g. delivering supervision and teaching on a regular basis). Reflecting on the impacts of your helping efforts, and taking action to balance self-care and other-care, can enable you to remain resilient and effective as a mentor. The ideas for mentee resilience in Chapter 10 are equally relevant to the mentor role.

A framework for reflective practice of mentoring – Gibbs' Reflective Cycle

Gibbs' Reflective Cycle (Gibbs, 1988) is a guide to reflecting on an encounter in order to make sense of what happened, learn from experience, and form commitments about future practice. Six categories of enquiry are part of the sequence, as shown in Figure 20. *See* Appendix K, p.246 for a worksheet based on Gibbs' Reflective Cycle, designed to guide reflective practice of mentoring.

Gibbs' Reflective Cycle is also relevant to the mentee's work as a doctor in practice, and may be used by the mentor to guide the mentee's reflective enquiry (*see* Chapter 4, pp.46–7, Appendix C, pp.201–4 and Appendix I, p.226.

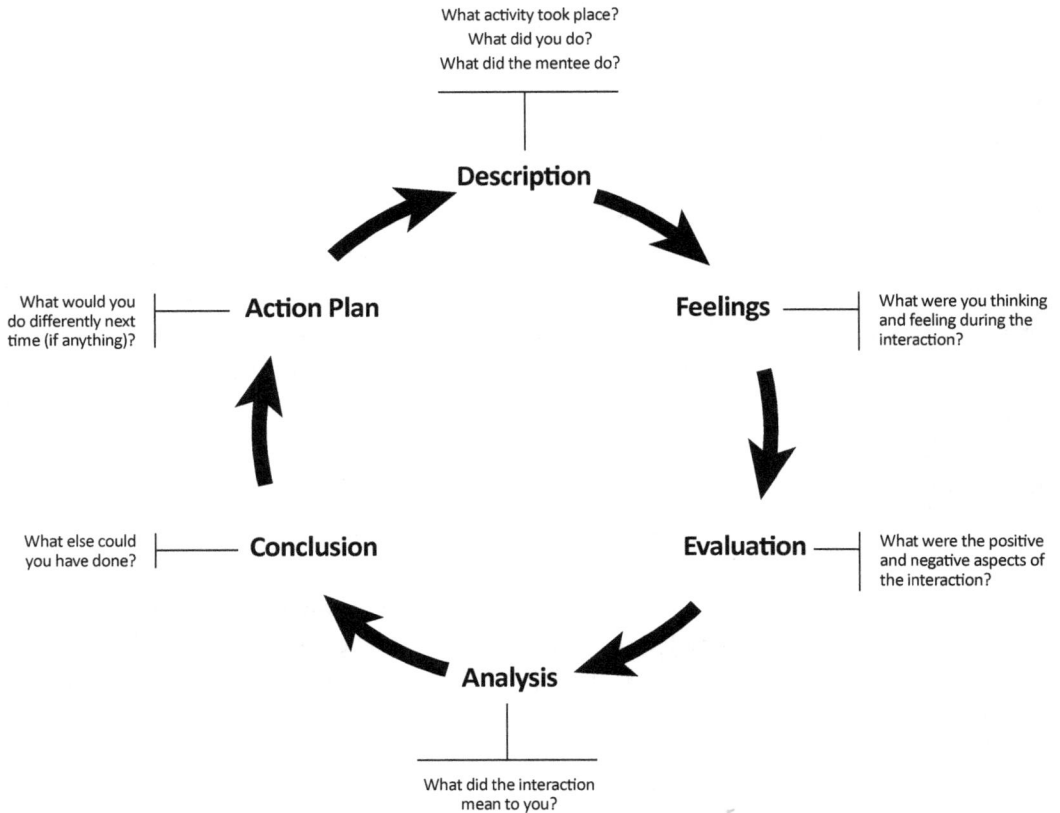

Figure 20. Using Gibbs' Reflective Cycle to guide the reflective practice of mentoring
Source: Gibbs (1988)

When to use reflective practice of mentoring

This tool is for **all** sessions.

Reflective practice has utility during a session for noticing what is taking place and what results are emerging, and making adjustments to your contributions as required in service of the mentee's goals. It also has utility after a session and at the conclusion of the partnership for thinking about the process that occurred, the outcomes, and your contributions to the partnership and process.

Pitfalls to avoid

- Not reflecting on mentoring practice
- Not reflecting on how past experiences may affect present mentoring practice
- Not examining experiences of difficult emotion elicited in mentoring
- Failing to adjust aspects of mentoring (e.g. mentoring activities) that are not helping the mentee to achieve their goals

3

Part Three:
Mentoring in practice

15. From theory to practice

Mentoring in summary

Mentoring is both a partnership and a process for development, and the work of mentoring is relational work and developmental work. Both mentor and mentee participate in this work. Intentional mentoring gives attention to the desired qualities of the mentoring partnership and process for development; ideally creating a **constructive partnership** and **productive process for development**, yielding developmental outcomes that are meaningful for the mentee. Table 13 provides a summary of key concepts in mentoring.

Table 13. Key concepts in mentoring

What mentoring is	What makes mentoring intentional	What a mentor does	What a mentee does	How to recognise value in mentoring	What a mentor and mentee pursue
A partnership of a mentor and a mentee	A constructive partnership	Relational work: Be trustworthy CARE – demonstrate commitment, accessibility, responsiveness and engagement	Relational work: Make and honour commitments Trust	Process evaluation	A safe space for the mentee
A process for the development of the mentee	A productive process	Developmental work: Positively influence the mentee's development as a doctor in practice	Developmental work: Develop as a doctor in practice, towards their aspirational state of development	Outcome evaluation	Transformation of the mentee

How to be an intentional mentor

Know your role

Your role is to do relational and developmental work with the mentee as agreed, incorporating support, challenge and facilitation, and to add structure to the mentoring. *See* Appendix D, pp.205–9 for a job description that summarises the mentor's work, knowledge, skills and attributes, and a resource that uses the metaphor of rock climbing training and the belayer role to illustrate mentoring and the mentor role.

Apply I-Mentor with the Cycle of Caring

The partnership and process aspects of mentoring are illustrated with the Model of Intentional Mentoring. Adding the Cycle of Caring (Skovholt, 2005) to the Model of Intentional Mentoring creates I-Mentor with the Cycle of Caring. This approach to the mentor role offers mentoring landmarks and signposts for mentoring practice. Empathic attachment, active involvement and felt separation are shown as the key stages. Within these stages of mentoring are a series of goal-directed interactions that assist the mentee to move towards or realise their aspirational state of development. Goal-directed interactions may contain episodes of brief intervention when accelerated progress is required.

Use the intentional mentor's toolkit

The intentional mentor aims to:

- build relationship and foster development in ways that are constructive and productive
- recognise and respond to the mentee's developmental needs for support, challenge and facilitation in service of their goals
- focus on doing more of what works, to assist the mentee to move towards their aspirational state of development.

Ten tools are central to this work: purposeful communication, partnership, goal-directed interaction, curriculum and performance standards, brief intervention, resilience work, career guidance, confidentiality, evaluation and reflective practice of mentoring. Table 14 presents a summary of the tools.

Table 14. A recap of the ten tools

TOOL	HOW TO USE THE TOOL	CASE STUDY REFERENCE
Purposeful communication (Tool #1) **A relating and developing tool** for achieving desired results in mentoring, based on listening, questioning and informing	Use active listening, questioning and informing to build relationship and foster development Use active listening, questioning and informing to support, challenge and facilitate Use agreed channels for communicating Be constructive	Conversation – Partnership set-up, *see* pp.140–3 Conversation – Learning knowledge, *see* pp.144–7 Conversation – Learning a skill, *see* pp.148–51 Conversation – Understanding and addressing performance problems that are complex, *see* pp.166–9
Partnership (Tool #2) **A connecting tool** for engaging with the mentee for the duration of mentoring and linking the mentee to the broader community of practice	Notice opportunities for forming a mentoring partnership Be aware of what you bring to mentoring Apply the Cycle of Caring Form a partnership using empathic attachment Collaborate using active involvement Part ways when the time is right, using felt separation	Conversation – Partnership set-up, *see* pp.140–3 Conversation – Learning a skill, *see* pp.148–51 Conversation – Concluding mentoring, *see* pp.173–8
Goal-directed Interaction (Tool #3) **A progress tool** for enhancing the mentee's success in setting and achieving goals, and realising their aspirational state of development	Assist the mentee to set goals Assist the mentee to achieve their goals Be guided by the mentee on the amount of structure to the interaction At the final session, part ways positively	Conversation – Partnership set-up, *see* pp.140–3 Conversation – Learning knowledge, *see* pp.144–7 Conversation – Learning a skill, *see* pp.148–51 Conversation – Improving performance of an essential task, *see* pp.169–71
Curriculum and performance standards (Tool #4) **A focusing tool** for identifying competency and performance requirements relevant to the mentee's practice	Identify the curriculum and performance standards most relevant to the mentee Be guided by curriculum and performance standards as a starting point for goal-directed interaction	Conversation – Partnership set-up, *see* pp.140–3 Conversation – Learning knowledge, *see* pp.144–7
Brief intervention (Tool #5) **An accelerating tool** for helping the mentee overcome obstacles and accelerate their progress towards goal achievement	Decide whether a brief intervention is warranted Offer the brief intervention with a clear rationale Notice the mentee's responses	Conversation – Learning clinical reasoning skills, *see* pp.151–5 Conversation – Insight, *see* pp.155–9

Resilience work (Tool #6) **A fortifying tool** for engaging with the mentee in relation to impacts of work and how to turn stress into adaptation	Work on stress management Work on energy management Work on self-preservation Use Purposeful communication (Tool #1), Partnership (Tool #2), Goal-directed interaction (Tool #3) and Confidentiality (Tool #8)	Conversation – Well-being, *see* pp.159–61 Conversation – Accountability, *see* pp.162–5 Conversation – Work-life balance, *see* pp.172–3 Conversation – Understanding and addressing performance problems that are complex, *see* pp.166–9
Career guidance (Tool #7) **A navigating tool** for orienting the mentee towards useful resources, actions and decisions in relation to career	Identify the mentee's vision of their place in the profession Connect the mentee to current and reliable resources Work collaboratively towards goal achievement	Conversation – Partnership set-up, *see* pp.140–3 Conversation – Work-life balance, *see* pp.172–3
Confidentiality (Tool #8) **A safety tool** for protection of confidential information shared during mentoring	Understand laws relevant to your mentoring practice Give the mentee an explanation of how your information management practices are law-abiding Discuss and decide whether to keep any records of mentoring Keep your promises to the mentee to protect their privacy	Conversation – Partnership set-up, *see* pp.140–3 Conversation – Well-being, *see* pp. 159–61 Conversation – Understanding and addressing performance problems that are complex, *see* pp.166–9
Evaluation (Tool #9) **A discovery tool** for identifying the mentee's response to mentoring and progress attributable to mentoring	Plan evaluation Notice what happened Notice what resulted Decide what to pay attention to as measures of success Use findings to improve future mentoring	Conversation – Accountability, *see* pp.162–5 Conversation – Concluding mentoring, *see* pp.173–8
Reflective practice of mentoring (Tool #10) **A self-monitoring tool** for learning about mentoring from experience	Reflect during each encounter with the mentee Reflect after each encounter with the mentee Evaluate your contribution to mentoring Determine actions to adjust your practice if required Join or form a mentoring community of practice Monitor the impacts of mentoring on you, and balance self-care and other-care	Not applicable

Troubleshooting

Part Two describes pitfalls to avoid in using each of the tools. Avoidance of the pitfalls decreases the chance of problems occurring during the course of mentoring, and increases the chance of the mentoring partnership and process being constructive and productive. However, problems may still arise in mentoring. Be prepared for this possibility. Remedial actions largely hinge on the use of Tool #1 Purposeful communication, with a focus on listening, questioning and informing to explore and understand the issues, and resolve the issues if possible. Mentoring is by nature a transitory partnership and parting ways is an option at all times. If a decision is made to conclude mentoring due to unresolved issues, it is preferable to conclude on a positive note, with respectful discussion of what worked, what did not work, and why.

16. Case study: Sam and Mikey

Applications of the intentional mentor's toolkit

In this chapter, mentor and mentee duo Sam and Mikey help to illustrate the mentoring partnership and process in true to life scenarios, and we highlight applications of the intentional mentor's toolkit. Tools are featured in chronological order by stage of the Cycle of Caring, that is, empathic attachment, active involvement and felt separation (Skovholt, 2005). In your mentoring practice, using these stages as landmarks for the course of mentoring enables you to participate in productive and constructive relational and developmental work, and deliver support, challenge and facilitation in a careful way.

Empathic attachment

Mikey's first day as a medical registrar

Mikey stepped into the lecture theatre for his orientation feeling more like it was his first day of high school than his first day as a medical registrar. The nervous energy from the morning was fast giving way to boredom as he was confronted with yet another workplace safety talk; this one was on how to lift a box without straining your back. He was hoping for the orientation to cover more things like 'How do I look confident when I have no idea what I'm doing?'

He chuckled to himself. He was told everyone felt this way. He looked around the room at all the others, putting on a brave face.

'Fake it 'til you make it,' he thought.

He had moved to this new city just last week, having received the good news of his acceptance onto the physician training program. He didn't start medical school planning to become a physician, but he had developed a love for it after his internship, and was affirmed by his senior colleagues. Still, he thought, a few rotations in medical specialties as a resident hardly prepares you for the responsibility of being a medical registrar – a role for which he felt woefully ill-equipped. He made a mental note to ask his friends in other professions if they felt the same way. The box-lifting lady handed over to someone he figured was a fire warden, because he was wearing a hard hat and brought in a fire extinguisher. Mikey wasn't sure how the hard hat helped one extinguish a fire. The morning groaned on.

The next session made his ears prick up. A confident-sounding, cheerful resident started talking about the hospital's mentoring program. Mikey was intrigued, the cheerful resident had a way of selling it that made it sound... well, helpful. Sign-ups were at morning tea, which was incidentally right after this session. Which was good. All of the mental box-lifting worked up an appetite.

When morning tea rolled around, it turned out that the mentors had actually come down to say hello. They seemed like nice people, genuinely interested to find out what the new batch of junior doctors were like. Mikey started talking to a general physician named Sam, who was perhaps ten years Mikey's senior. Sam liked cycling and golf, which they bonded over, since Mikey was a road cyclist, and he thoroughly enjoyed Happy Gilmore.

When the announcement came that morning tea was over, and the next session was starting, Mikey quickly filled out the mentoring sign-up form. Who knows, he thought. Maybe it will help.

Conversation – Partnership set-up

Mikey wandered down the corridors of his new hospital. A week in, and he was still having difficulty finding his way around the rabbit warren. He was on his way to meet Sam again; the mentor he had been paired with through the hospital's mentoring program. Sam seemed like a good person to learn from, and they got along quite well on orientation day, so he was looking forward to seeing what a mentoring partnership might bring.

He stopped and asked for directions from one of the administration staff, who directed him further down the corridor and to the left. He followed the directions and found the door to Sam's office open. He peered in and saw Sam sitting at a desk in a fairly modest office. There were a few journals and textbooks on the shelf, a desktop computer on the desk, and a few pictures of family hung on the wall. Fairly standard, but neat and tidy.

Sam looked up from his desk as Mikey tapped politely on the open door. He stood up and smiled, and offered his hand to Mikey.

'Mikey,' he said, shaking his hand firmly. 'Great to see you again.'

'Likewise,' said Mikey, 'Thanks for making the time.'

Sam gestured to a seat, which Mikey took. 'No problem. This is only my second year as a mentor in the program, so putting my cards on the table – we'll be learning how to do this together, and I probably won't have all the answers!'

'Don't worry, I've never had a mentor before, so I guess we'll just have to see how it goes,' said Mikey, secretly a little relieved that there was some flexibility here. 'How do these things usually work?'

'Well, it's really up to you,' said Sam. 'I'm here to be a sounding board, a listening ear, and to help you get where you want to go – we want you to develop. The whole idea of the partnership is to be intentional, but flexible. The first thing to do is to figure out what you want to get out of the next year or two here. Then we can establish some goals, and figure out how we can achieve them. Along the way, we troubleshoot.'

'Okay, great,' said Mikey. 'I haven't really thought about my training in that way before. I guess I just thought that developing as a doctor was something you got by osmosis.'

'Well, to a degree, it is,' agreed Sam. 'We probably learn that way more than we realise. But being intentional and goal-focused is far more effective for achieving specific results. So let me ask you this: what do you hope to achieve in the next two years whilst you're here with us?'

'I guess I haven't really thought about it. Learn how to be a decent medical registrar is probably a good starting place. Passing my exams next year would be great, too. I'm also pretty keen to try my hand at some research; I really only have a few case reports to my name, and would really like to get more involved in this area,' pondered Mikey.

'Good start. Might I suggest that you also consider your life outside of work too? I've seen a few registrars burn out from working too hard. It can help to make it a specific goal,' suggested Sam.

'Yeah, good thinking. I've seen it go badly, too,' said Mikey.

Sam replied, 'Ok, that's a good start. We have four goals: improve your general competency as a physician, pass your exams, publish a paper and look after yourself! Let's just start to tackle the first one for today, and then we can discuss the others the next time we get together.'

'Sure,' said Mikey. 'Competency. Sounds important!'

Sam chuckled. 'It does. Let's make the goal more specific. Is there anything you want to look at in particular?'

'Well, I guess the thing that worries me the most is knowing how to get myself out of trouble in an emergency, like a code blue or MET call. Emergencies can escalate very quickly, often before you have the chance to get the consultant if it's after hours,' said Mikey, with a slightly worried look.

'Sure,' replied Sam. 'It takes a few months before you get comfortable there. It will be a few months before we put you on after hours by yourself, so that gives us a good timeframe. Let's frame it this way, and write it down – Mikey wants to be sufficiently competent at managing medical emergencies so as to practice comfortably without immediate supervision within 3 months. What do you think?'

Mikey thought well of it, so wrote it down word for word.

'Ok, so the next step is to figure out where you're at now. Have you had much experience with codes?' asked Sam.

'Only as a resident,' replied Mikey. 'Mostly putting in drips, taking blood gases and the like. I can do CPR pretty well, but I don't really know how to think clearly when everything is going wrong. I'm not sure how to run the team in that situation. Also, I'm not sure I'm up to scratch with the most recent guidelines.'

'That's really good insight, Mikey. You've identified two main things to work on – knowledge of the guidelines, and calm thinking and communication during an emergency. The next question is; how do we work on these things? Do you know of any resources that might help you?'

'Do we have a simulation lab? I'd love to try that.'

'Great idea,' replied Sam. 'Might I also suggest you have a look at the most recent Australian Resuscitation Guidelines? It will be worthwhile before we get you up to the sim lab. The sim lab here is great; they will give you as many sessions as you need.'

'That would be excellent. Thanks Sam.'

'No problem. Now we have a goal, we have assessed the reality of where you're at, we've thought about the obstacles and we have a way forward. What do you think?' asked Sam.

'That's great. Really. Thanks. I'm feeling much more comfortable just having an idea about how to tackle things. This has been really helpful.'

'I'm glad, Mikey. Oh, and one more thing. Just to let you know that anything you share here stays between us – it's all confidential. I won't share anything with anyone unless there's a legal issue that I'm bound to disclose. Otherwise, this is a safe space. Now, I'll let you get back to work. Let's catch up again in four weeks to see how you're tracking with that,' suggested Sam.

Mikey stood to leave, and shook Sam's hand firmly. 'Thanks again, I really appreciate it.'

Scenario precis

Mikey moves to a new town and a new hospital to start physician training. He goes through orientation and hears about the mentoring program, and links in with Sam. This is, of course, only one way that a mentoring partnership can begin. Many may find it preferable to commence a mentoring partnership out of a pre-existing relationship. Whatever the avenue into mentoring the initial conversations are crucial. We see Sam and Mikey begin to form a bond over their mutual interests during the empathic attachment stage; though of course, you will see such attachment continue to develop over the ensuing partnership.

The first formal mentoring conversation commences the active involvement stage. Note that the conversation is intentionally goal-directed and focused on development. One of Mikey's goals is to publish a paper, one is to pass his exams. In this short conversation, Sam uses many tools: Purposeful communication (Tool #1), Partnership (Tool #2), Goal-directed interaction (Tool #3), Curriculum and performance standards (Tool #4), Career guidance (Tool #7) and Confidentiality (Tool # 8).

Active involvement

Conversation – Learning knowledge

Mikey sat at the back of the room during the handover meeting after what was evidently a long night shift. The night registrar, the one doing the talking, was one year his senior and was sitting her exams soon. As he listened to her talk, he was struck by a bolt of fear. She just knew so much. How did she get to know that much? Is that the kind of knowledge you need to have to pass the exam? If so, Mikey was in trouble. He was planning to sit his exams in the following year, so he had a bit over twelve months to prepare. That was a long time. But it was also a lot to know.

He had coasted a bit during medical school. He was a crammer. He did okay, finished somewhere in the middle of the class. But he never really learned how to manage his time. Discipline was lacking. Middle of the class was okay when ninety-five percent of the class passed. Middle of the class was not okay when only fifty percent passed, as was the case with most post-graduate exams. He had no idea where to start. He needed some help.

Soon the meeting drew to a close, and the tired night registrar wandered out the door, presumably to collapse into the nearest bed. Mikey saw Sam leaving the meeting and jogged to catch up.

'Sam,' he said when he was only a few feet behind.

Sam turned and smiled. 'Mikey, how are you? Good to see you.'

'Sam, can I ask you something?'

'Sure, what's on your mind?'

'You know how we mentioned exams as one of my goals for my time here? Well, I've been freaking out a bit; I've got no idea where to get started. Can you give me some pointers?'

'Sure thing,' replied Sam. 'Have you got 20 minutes?'

'Yeah, I guess. Clinic doesn't start until nine.'

'Great. Come to my office, I've got my old notes and study schedule on my desktop.'

They tracked down the corridor to Sam's office. Mikey again noted Sam's understated and tidy office space. Sam was an organised person. Mikey was...not. The closest thing Mikey had to an office was the desk in his bedroom, and it got decluttered about once every 6 months when the pile of papers was about to topple over. Mikey took an offered seat across from Sam, who got to work waking up his computer.

'What do you know about the exams, Mikey?' Sam asked.

'Not much. Just what you hear from the senior registrars. I gather they're hard.'

'That they are,' Sam chuckled. 'What kind of studier are you?'

'A bad one,' Mikey sighed. 'I mostly crammed in medical school. I'm more of an on-the-job learner. But that's not going to help me pass a written exam.'

'Well, it can. We just have to find a way to make it work for you. What kind of obstacles do you see between you and passing the exam?'

'Knowledge, or lack thereof. I was listening to Kirsty in the handover meeting today. She just knows so much. I don't know where she finds the time or energy to fit it all in her head, working 60 hours a week, on nights half the time, you know? I mean, short of giving up your life completely for a year, how do you tackle it?' Mikey asked.

'No way around it,' replied Sam. 'It's hard work. But if you are sensible and you pace yourself, you can do it. And you don't need to give up your life. Well, at least not completely.'

'Right – but where do I start?'

'Well, let's make a plan. Your goal is to acquire the knowledge you need to pass the exam this time next year, right? So all we need to figure out is where you are now, and how we get you from here to there.' Sam gestured with hands, making a line between two points on the invisible timeline of Mikey's life.

'Well, that's easy. I'm not really anywhere. I know a bit of practical stuff, but not much to help me pass. In fact, I don't even know the curriculum,' exclaimed Mikey.

'That's easy to fix and a good place to start. Now, what are the other obstacles?'

'Time, I suppose. We are busy, you know, we work hard. I'm generally pretty tired when I get home. I just want to watch the game or catch up with friends. How do we overcome that?' asked Mikey.

'A few ways. A timetable helps – there's actually more time in the day than you think there is. There is time that can be redeemed. Also, a study group helps to share the load. Have you given any thought to that?'

'Not really. I know Tom and Bec want to sit next year as well, and we get along pretty well. Maybe we could form a group,' Mikey pondered.

'Great,' said Sam. 'So our goal is for you to acquire enough knowledge to pass the exam this time next year. At the moment, we haven't really started, and you've identified your study technique and lack of time as potential obstacles. We're going to try and overcome this in several ways. First, you're going to write down a timetable of your week, and set aside five hours per week to study. That will have to increase, but let's start low and go slow. Then you can approach Tom and Bec about a study group – I suggest you get started by looking into the curriculum and coming up with a year-long plan to get through the material; remember to leave some time for revision. I'll email you my old schedule – it was a few years ago now but it will be something to work off. Then we can meet again and check with how you're going. Do you think three weeks will be enough time?'

'Should be. Chase me up if I haven't got it together by then.'

'Will do, Mikey. Also, can I give you one piece of advice when it comes to studying for post-grad exams?' asked Sam.

'Please – I'm all ears,' said Mikey.

'Don't get too caught up with the time you spend studying. The five hours a week is really just to dedicate some space. Set a goal for what you want to learn in a session, not on how long that session should be. If you've been sitting there for an hour and haven't learned anything because you're too tired, the best thing you can do is go to bed and try again in the morning. Knowledge passes the exam. Not time spent trying to acquire it. Make sure you structure in a contingency plan in case something happens prior to the exam, like a family emergency where you have to have a few weeks off. Make sure you can afford that time.'

'Thanks – I'll remember that,' said Mikey.

'Great. You better get to clinic. When you get a no-show, use that time to look up something about the case you just saw. It will help.'

'Will do. See you in three weeks. Thanks, Sam.'

'My pleasure, Mikey.'

Scenario precis

This conversation covers a topic relevant to all junior doctors: how to acquire the necessary knowledge to perform at a satisfactory level in the medical profession. Although the vehicle for the knowledge acquisition in this context is exam pressure, the same principles can be applied to those who are not sitting exams but who require further knowledge to perform competently.

Again, we can see Purposeful communication (Tool #1) and Goal-directed interaction (Tool #3) at play here. Firstly, there is a deliberate recognition of where Mikey is currently – his 'book knowledge' is lacking. Secondly, where Mikey needs to be is defined – he requires enough knowledge to pass his exam. Lastly, what Mikey requires to achieve his goal is clearly articulated, along with recognition of the barriers he will face.

Note also that the goals (both short and long term) set are SMART goals.
Specific: The goal is to acquire knowledge needed to pass the exam.
Measurable: Ultimately the knowledge gain will be measured by passing the exam, however there are short term goals that are easily measured too; formation of a study group, for example.
Assignable: Sam and Mikey each take on responsibilities related to Mikey's goal; Mikey commits to setting aside five hours per week of dedicated study time and organising a study group, while Sam commits to sharing a study schedule and tips based on his own experiences.
Realistic: Sam has twelve months to prepare for the exam, and although daunted by the task, he is aware that it is a realistic goal as others including Sam have passed the exam; Sam uses some of his past experience with the exam to add some reality to the situation for Mikey and reassure that the goal is achievable.
Time related: The short term goal of forming a study group has a timeframe of three weeks and the ultimate goal of passing the exam has a longer timeframe of over twelve months.

Curriculum and performance standards (Tool #4) is another tool Sam uses in this conversation. Sam suggests the training curriculum as an appropriate resource for producing a study timetable. Sam and Mikey are in the same field, so Sam has a working knowledge and familiarity with the curriculum. However, this will not be the case for many mentoring partnerships. Mentors should familiarise themselves (at least conceptually) with the curriculum of their mentees, however a detailed knowledge of their curriculum is usually not necessary.

Conversation – Learning a skill

Mikey was a bit frustrated with himself. He had missed a lumbar puncture earlier in the day, and had to hand over to his consultant to finish. He didn't like doing that. He considered himself quite good with his hands, but for some reason he just couldn't find the right spot. It was distressing for the patient and frustrating for him.

It was still fairly early in his training. He had only really seen lumbar punctures done in the past; he hadn't done any himself. This was his first solo attempt. And it hadn't gone well. Of course, he was going to have to learn, because as a medical registrar the lumbar puncture was a frequent procedure, and often very important.

Then a thought cut across his mind. How do you actually learn a procedure? It seemed different to just learning facts. You can know exactly how to do a procedure and not be able to do it well. He thought about the old mantra, 'see one, do one, teach one.' Well and good, he thought. But not exactly useful when you failed at the 'do one' part. He really needed another way.

He set off to the medical offices, hoping to run into Sam and ask him some advice. As it happened, Sam was sitting in his office, door open with an imposing pile of paperwork on the desk. Sam heard Mikey at the door, looked up and smiled.

'Mikey, hi. How are you?' Sam asked.

'Not bad, Sam. At least I'm not about to drown in paperwork!' He joked.

'Ahh, yes,' sighed Sam, 'You think the paperwork slows down the more senior you get, but trust me, it gets worse!'

'Not what I was hoping for! Mind if I interrupt for a minute or two?'

'Please do. What's on your mind?' asked Sam.

'I need a bit of advice. I'm a medical registrar and I can't do a lumbar puncture solo yet. I really need to get it sorted out! I'm on nights for the first time in a few weeks, and I won't have a consultant there to bail me out. What if I need to do one?' asked Mikey.

'It's certainly an important procedure,' agreed Sam. 'And doing it safely and competently is an essential part of your training. How are you at procedures in general?'

'I thought I was pretty good at them. I've done a few abdominal paracenteses without incident, and I can hardly remember the last time I couldn't get an IV cannula in.'

'Well, LP's are really just a variation on a theme. How did you learn how to put in a drip?' asked Sam.

'I really can't remember,' replied Mikey. 'I guess you just start doing it, and eventually it's muscle memory.'

'That's partly right, I think. But you've probably forgotten all the hard work you did and all the frustration the first time you missed an IV. The majority of the learning happens at the start. If you'll excuse the colloquialism, it's like riding a bike. Not in the sense that it's easy to come back to after a long time off; though that's somewhat true. In the sense that you do a lot of learning by falling off, until one day you don't fall off anymore,' said Sam.

'Right,' said Mikey, 'so how do I do enough 'bike riding' that I don't fall off anymore?'

'It's different for everyone, but if you're a natural proceduralist hopefully it won't take too long. The first thing I'd do is try and unlearn any bad habits. You've probably seen a bunch of people do them – and everyone does them differently, right?'

'Right. I don't even know whether you do them with the patient sitting or lying,' said Mikey.

'It doesn't really matter which way you choose, but pick whichever way works for you and stick to it. I personally prefer lying down, because you can check the opening pressure and it's usually more comfortable for the patient. But sitting up gives you slightly better symmetry. Whatever works. But what I definitely would do is start by watching a good video a few times. The New England Journal of Medicine procedural videos are excellent – start there, memorise the steps,' suggested Sam.

'Okay, that seems easy enough,' said Mikey.

'Next, you really do just need to practice. It's tricky because there's no simulator, and you can't just practice on your colleagues like you can with IV lines! So you need to be able to hone your skills on patients who need it done. Where do you think you might be able to find them?'

'I suppose places where they're done all the time. Maybe in Emergency, or neurology,' thought Mikey.

'Haematology as well, they do a lot for intrathecal chemotherapy. Why don't you approach your colleagues? Often the neurologists have patients coming in to the day unit to have an LP – I'm sure they would be delighted to give you some of their work!' exclaimed Sam.

'That's a good idea. It's a slightly more predictable environment than emergency,' said Mikey.

'Absolutely. Make sure you start out with technically easy ones first. Get your confidence up. Get your position and anatomical landmarks fixed in your mind. Then slowly work up to more technically difficult patients,' suggested Sam.

'That's a good idea. The patient today was quite tricky – they had had back surgery before and they weren't able to get into a good position,' said Mikey.

'That's a trap! Don't try running before you can walk.'

'Good advice,' said Mikey.

'So I'm just going to recap. At the moment, you can't do a lumbar puncture. You want to be able to perform one safely and independently by the time your night shifts come around next month. You're going to achieve this by watching a procedural video, then approaching your colleagues for real-time practice under supervision. I can put you in touch with some of the neurologists who would be willing to help if you like?'

'Thanks Sam, that would be great. Now, I should let you get back to your paperwork!'

'I think I'd rather have a lumbar puncture. But you're most welcome. Let me know how you go,' said Sam.

'Will do, thanks,' said Mikey as he left, feeling far more optimistic about the way forward.

Scenario precis

In this scenario, Sam uses Purposeful communication (Tool #1) and Goal-directed interaction (Tool #3) to facilitate Mikey's learning of a skill – lumbar puncture. The skill is procedural, but not all skills are procedural, such as clinical reasoning skills (covered in the next conversation). Learning a procedural skill requires a significant investment of time and effort from both the mentee and the mentor due to the repetition and feedback involved. As the mentee's competence develops over time, the developmental work requires Partnership (Tool #2).

Note in this scenario that Sam is invested in the outcome, going out of his way to ensure that Mikey has adequate exposure to opportunities to learn the new skill. This is one way that a mentor is different from an educator; a mentor goes the extra step of ensuring that the desired outcome is achieved.

Mentors in different fields to mentees will require a more dynamic approach to facilitating learning of a skill that is outside the field of the mentor, as the mentor will not be the one directly teaching the skill. In this circumstance, the role of the mentor is to oversee the development and offer guidance about how to proceed further, potentially engaging a third party to invest in the process.

Conversation – Learning clinical reasoning skills

It was the end of a busy clinic, and Mikey's last patient was a 48-year-old woman with the worst luck. She had endometrial cancer when she was 40, and then had surgery and chemotherapy and was cured. Eight years later she developed rectal bleeding. A GP visit, and a colonoscopy and biopsy later, Mikey had to tell her she now had colon cancer. Some people just had the worst luck.

As was the procedure at the clinic, when he wasn't one hundred per cent sure what to do next he left the patient in her clinic room and went to wait for the consultant. She was a bit shell-shocked, so he asked one of the clinic nurses to sit in with her whilst she waited. It was Sam's clinic today, and he had just finished with his last patient when Mikey knocked.

'Mikey,' Sam said, 'How are you? Are you done?'

'Almost,' Mikey said. 'I just have one question for you about the lady I'm seeing at the moment.' He told Sam the sad story. 'I'm just wondering how we go about staging her.'

'Interesting case,' Sam said, deep in thought. 'Before we get to the staging, I'm just going to make sure we haven't closed off prematurely here. Does she have any family history?'

'Ahh, forgot to ask,' said Mikey, annoyed at himself. He still made silly mistakes or omissions like this on a semi-regular basis. 'Also, what does it mean to close prematurely?

Sam recognised his annoyance. 'Premature closure is when you assume you have the diagnosis correct, such that you don't entertain any other possibilities. Why did I ask about family history?'

Mikey thought for a moment. 'Presumably you were thinking of some kind of familial syndrome.'

'Yes, that's right. Do you know of any?' Sam asked.

'Well, in med school they mentioned the BRCA genes for breast cancer, and a few others. I can't recall,' answered Mikey, trying desperately to conjure up an image of his genetics lectures from five years previous.

'I'm thinking particularly of a syndrome called HNPCC, or Lynch syndrome. Heard of it?'

'It rings a bell,' said Mikey, but he couldn't figure out why.

'It's a familial cancer syndrome. There's an error in a gene encoding DNA mismatch repair. The two most common cancers are colon and endometrial, but there are other cancers too, like ovarian and other GIT cancers. It's dominantly inherited, hence my question about family history.'

'Right,' said Mikey. 'I guess these are things that you just have to know, right?'

'Well, yes and no,' replied Sam. 'Knowing about HNPCC certainly helps, and you certainly should know about it. Look up the Amsterdam criteria. But knowing about HNPCC wasn't the whole reason I took an interest. Doesn't something about this case strike you as unusual?'

'Well, I guess so,' said Mikey. 'She's pretty young for two cancers, particularly cancers that are usually found in people who are over fifty or sixty. I just thought she was unlucky.'

'No doubt she is unlucky. But we should figure out if she is genetically unlucky or just plain old unlucky. Why do you think that's important?' probed Sam.

'Good question,' said Mikey, giving himself time to think. 'I guess it's of relevance to her family members, they might need to be screened.'

'Good,' said Sam. 'And for her too. She still has other organs that can get cancer.'

'Wow. Okay. How do you think of all this stuff?'

'Well, partly it's just experience, but there are ways that you can train yourself to think. The first principle is thoroughness. You missed the family history; that's okay, we all forget sometimes. But there is a reason why it's part of a routine history – it's a safety net. If she had told you that her dad died of colon cancer at 45, you probably would have thought something's up, right?'

'Right,' Mikey agreed.

'The second principle is pattern recognition. Now that does come with experience. Now that you've seen bowel and endometrial cancer in one patient in real life, you won't forget it.'

'Ha. Hopefully,' Mikey exclaimed.

'You won't. Trust me. Third, use some reductionism. When you get that little niggle in the back of your mind that something isn't quite right, you have to go back to first principles. I know that oncology is a subspecialty you haven't done yet, but think about what could tie the two together? Ockham's razor, right?'

'Right. A unifying diagnosis is more likely than two separate ones,' Mikey recalled.

'The final thing you need to remember is an assessment of risk. That helps you to determine what you do next. If the risk was lower, for example, if she was eighty and had no family history, then further testing probably wouldn't be warranted. But the risk for her is quite high, and the risk involved with missing the diagnosis is also substantial – her children, her siblings, should all be tested if this turns out to be HNPCC.'

'Which sounds pretty likely at this stage,' said Mikey.

'Well, maybe,' Sam replied. 'But we should check. If the test turns out negative, we will have to re-evaluate our hypothesis. We might find that you were right all along and she's just unlucky. Let's refer her to genetics and to the oncologists and surgeons for more work-up. I'll come meet her.'

'Thanks, Sam. I appreciate it.'

'No problem. Just remember your clinical reasoning tools: thoroughness, pattern recognition, reductionistic thinking, risk assessment and re-evaluation when you get new information. Your knowledge is the cherry on top – knowing you need to look is most of the battle.'

'Great. I'll remember that.'

Scenario precis

Clinical reasoning is not something that can be distilled onto a few pages, nor is it something that can be taught in five minutes following clinic. It takes years, and it's difficult, and even experienced clinicians get it wrong sometimes.

However, that is not to say that learning clinical reasoning happens passively. It is still a profoundly active process. For learning of this nature, Brief intervention (Tool #5) is useful. In this case, Sam offers Mikey a brief intervention in order help Mikey develop. Note that the brief intervention is opportunistic – it turns an everyday scenario into a development opportunity, which is of great advantage to most time-poor mentors and mentees.

First, Sam recognises that there are two major issues with Mikey's approach. He has demonstrated both a lack of knowledge of familial cancer syndromes, and a lack of thoroughness in his clinical history. In this case, had Mikey displayed either knowledge or thoroughness, he would have been alerted to the diagnosis. This is why medical students are taught to be extremely thorough in their history and examination, as they lack the necessary knowledge to be more succinct.

Sam also introduces four other concepts that can alert a clinician to a potentially serious diagnostic error: pattern recognition, reductionist thinking, risk assessment and re-evaluation. All of these processes act together to help make a diagnosis and a management plan, and when all of them are employed they act like layers of Swiss cheese. The more layers you have, the less likely it is that the 'hole' in that particular area will line up with the 'holes' in all the other areas.

Whilst Sam introduces all of these concepts to Mikey in the brief intervention, it is unlikely that Mikey will have grasped them all immediately. This active process ideally occurs over a long period of time, where individual skills are honed. Knowledge and thoroughness are focused on here, with an expectation that the others would be worked on at a later date when an opportunity presents.

Conversation – Insight

Mikey was tired. Not gee-I-could-go-for-a-nap tired. This was the kind of weariness that seeps into your bones. The kind that meant you had to think – hard – about even the most routine tasks that you ordinarily performed via reflex.

He was finishing up his last of seven night shifts. They had been busy. No major disasters, but no sleep either. Compiling his fatigue was his inability to sleep well during the day.

His circadian rhythm did not like being disturbed. He was one of those people who needed his bed, his pillow, and a dark, quiet, cool room to sleep well. He envied those people who could fall asleep on planes and trains and buses. He couldn't. He couldn't even fall asleep in a lecture.

He'd seen two nursing shift changes this shift. First the evening handed over to the night staff, and about an hour ago the night staff handed over to the day. Now the residents were diligently filing in, getting lists prepared and ready for the day's work. He walked past the nurses station on his way to the handover meeting. A nursing student stopped him along the way.

'Mikey,' she said, 'Mrs Buchanan in bed 6 is vomiting after the morphine we gave her. Can you write her up something?'

'Ah, sure,' said Mikey, wanting to be helpful, but also wishing she had of asked one of the people who walked in five minutes ago, and not the guy who looked like the walking dead. 'How is her pain?' he asked.

'Much better,' she replied.

Mikey took the chart and wrote Metoclopramide, 10mg, IV, stat. The nursing student thanked him and walked back into room 6.

He turned to walk towards the handover meeting when Sam walked in, coffee in hand. He seemed to have that odd combination of always looking busy, but not looking flustered. Sam saw Mikey and walked over.

'Looks like you need one of these!' Sam said with a slight raise of his coffee cup.

'I think I'm beyond that. What I need is one of those,' replied Mikey, pointing into an open room that had an empty bed in it.

'I hear you. Let's get to the handover meeting so you can get home to sleep,' said Sam.

They turned to walk to the handover room. As they were about to get to the door, Mikey was stopped as someone called his name from behind. He turned to see the senior nurse for Mrs Buchanan walking up to him, chart in hand.

'Mrs Buchanan is allergic to metoclopramide. She had an occulogyric crisis last time. You need to write her something else,' she said.

Mikey felt his heart sink. That could have been serious. He looked at the chart. Right there, clear as day in the allergy section, it was written Maxolon. The nursing student probably didn't realise metoclopramide and Maxolon were the same thing. But he knew. And he should have checked. Thank God for experienced nurses, he thought.

'Oh, man. That was a bad miss. Thanks for picking that up,' he said, as he crossed out his old order, and wrote a new one for ondansetron.

She thanked him, took the chart and turned back to the room.

Sam could see the distress on Mikey's face. He knew Mikey was usually very careful. Carelessness was not really an issue for him.

'Mikey,' said Sam, 'We all make mistakes like that. Every doctor has done it. That's why we have multiple checks in place – the system is there to save you.'

'Yeah, I know. But I hate it when I do something like that. I always check for allergies. Why didn't I check this time? It would have been serious,' exclaimed Mikey, pinching the bridge of his nose in frustration.

'It was a near miss. But that's why the system is there. It is, however, a good learning point,' said Sam.

'How so?'

'It teaches you something about recognising barriers, and being aware of your shortcomings. In this case, the barrier is tiredness. When you're this tired, even small, routine things become difficult. You forget to do things you would normally do. It happens to everyone. What you need to be aware of is how tiredness affects you, and put some safety nets in place when you know you're not at your best. For example, I will often ask a colleague to check my orders when I know I'm not thinking clearly. Just add that extra layer of safety by letting them know that you're not 100%.'

'So I should just be more careful? I don't know – I'm not sure I can trust myself to do that all the time,' said Mikey.

'Well, it's not just about being more careful Mikey. But you're right about not trusting yourself when you're not at your best. It's awareness. A useful acronym is HALT – Hungry, Angry, Late, Tired. All of these things impair your judgment. It's going to happen to you plenty of times in the future; when you get called in the middle of the night for an emergency, for example. You need to be aware that you aren't going to be as sharp as you would be in the middle of the day, and let your colleagues know – give them permission – to double-check your orders. Better awareness leads to better safety. Trust me – you'll see the sense of it after some sleep!'

'Thanks, Sam.'

'That's okay. Now let's get to the meeting so that you can get home.'

Scenario precis

This conversation canvasses an all-too-familiar situation for doctors. The rates of medication errors in hospitals are enormous. Although most of them are trivial, a significant proportion of them can lead to serious consequences.

With this Brief intervention (Tool #5), Sam teaches Mikey the concept of awareness. Gone are the days (thankfully) when doctors were seen as infallible creatures whose orders were not to be questioned. However, pockets of this kind of attitude remain in some institutions, and the concept of awareness helps us to combat this. Doctors must be aware of their own shortcomings and biases, whether transient (such as tiredness) or more permanent traits, and should invite help when required.

Again, it should be noted that the brief intervention occurs in a routine daily scenario.

In this particular circumstance, it needs to be handled in a sensitive manner: Mikey has made a mistake, and he is tired. He would be feeling vulnerable. He is already well aware of his mistake, and does not need it pointed out to him further. Sam's response is to turn the scenario into an opportunity for development. Disciplinary action is necessary in some cases, particularly if the error is deliberate, malicious or unprofessional. However, Sam makes the assessment that in this circumstance no disciplinary action is required; what's required is development.

Sam's response to Mikey's error is empathic. The idea is not to make Mikey feel bad about his error, but rather to help Mikey learn from his error. The response is developmental, not destructive. It builds up, it does not belittle. It recognises that humans (even doctors!) are fallible, and that systems are in place to restrict human error. Gibbs' Reflective Cycle (Gibbs, 1988) is at work in the conversation when Sam explores what happened, the meaning of the experience, and what Mikey will do differently in the future. The response does not endorse carelessness, but rather emphasises the importance of self-awareness, and careful consideration of even trivial tasks that may have serious consequences.

Conversation – Well-being

Mikey wasn't himself. He thought he was going really well, was starting to feel confident. He was starting to feel at home as a medical registrar. Then it happened. Out of the blue. One of his young patients died of a pulmonary embolism. Just like that. They knew the diagnosis. They had done all the right things. The patient seemed fine. Then, bang. It just happened. She arrested all of a sudden, despite being on the right treatment.

It wasn't supposed to work like that. He had gone back over the scenario many times in his head. What if he had have made the diagnosis a bit earlier? What if he had thrombolysed when she was in Emergency? What if he had given IV heparin instead of subcutaneous enoxaparin? Around and around in circles.

He had been assured many times by everyone involved that she received appropriate care. 'Gold standard,' even. But that didn't seem to make it easier when Mikey and his consultant had to explain to her family that she died suddenly and unexpectedly.

Everyone in the department knew what had happened, and Sam could see Mikey was struggling with it, so he brought him in to his office to check in.

'Mikey,' said Sam, 'You've had a rough week. How are you doing?'

Mikey looked blank. 'I feel terrible,' he said in a matter-of-fact tone. 'It shouldn't happen like that. We did everything right. When you do everything right, things are supposed to go well, right?'

Sam gave Mikey a soft smile, and let him continue.

'I mean, I think we did everything right. I've been over it dozens of times in my head. She was treated according to the guidelines. Why did it go so badly?'

'Do you think you did anything wrong?' probed Sam.

'No, well, I don't think so. Not wrong, per se. But I do wonder if I could have done anything better. You know, something that could have made a difference,' replied Mikey.

'I know how you feel. I remember a similar case a few years ago. It was awful. A young guy died from infective endocarditis that he got from a thorn prick on the finger whilst gardening. We tried everything, but he just kept going downhill,' Sam sympathized.

'How'd you deal with it?' asked Mikey.

'Probably the first thing was to get realistic about what we actually can do, and more importantly what we can't do. We are better at making that distinction when people are elderly or have chronic health problems, but some people are just plain unlucky. We just can't reverse what's gone wrong sometimes,' Sam offered.

'But surely we could have done something else? Thrombolysed, or put in an IVC filter?' asked Mikey.

'Sure, you could have – but you made the right decision with the information you had at the time. Besides, you know the evidence, and you know that it probably wouldn't have made a difference. She was unlucky. These are the clinical scenarios that we have to deal with. We don't have a crystal ball – you just have to accept that we do all we can, with the best of intentions. Mostly we win, but often we lose. It's the reality of our job. It's dreadful. But it is what it is.'

'Right – but how do you handle it? You know, emotionally?' asked Mikey.

'It's not easy. Talking helps. Leaning on your colleagues and friends. Talk to the hospital counselling service if you need to. But I found the most effective thing was to think about all the people that we have helped. That helps me to stay resilient, without becoming uncaring,' Sam offered.

'That's helpful, thanks,' said Mikey.

'That's okay. Listen, this isn't going to get better straight away. It's going to take time. Take whatever time you need, and let me know if you're struggling. Maybe you need a few days off to do something you enjoy. Do you think you need some formal counselling?'

'I think I'm okay for now. Let me process for another day or two, and then I'll come back to you,' suggested Mikey.

'Sounds good, Mikey.'

Scenario precis

In this scenario, Mikey deals with the difficult situation of having a patient die unexpectedly. This is a common scenario in hospitals, and among doctors, reactions are diverse.

It is important to note that in this scenario, Sam is not operating as Mikey's counsellor. He recognises that there may be a need for formal counselling at some point. Sam is acting here as Mikey's mentor and is predominantly using Resilience work (Tool #6) to ensure Mikey is looking after himself. The medical profession is high-stress and high-stakes. It is impossible to remove all factors that might impact on a doctor's well-being, so developing coping mechanisms and resilience is paramount.

Sam does three things that are of critical importance to foster Mikey's resilience. Firstly, he knows Mikey well enough (i.e. his 'baseline') to identify when there is a problem. This is not always the easiest thing to do, as some people are extremely good at hiding their difficulties. Occasional probing questions to detect well-being problems are useful when the problem is not obvious.

Secondly, he empathises with a story of his own. This involves Confidentiality (Tool #8), as Sam makes a considered decision to share some confidential information of his own within the boundaries of the partnership.

Lastly, he offers advice to Mikey to help him through the situation. This advice takes two forms; professional and personal. The professional advice is how to develop resilience through these common workplace problems. The personal advice is about having some down time, and seeking counselling if necessary. This may seem to be an obvious suggestion, but a healthy home life is, for most people, essential to the type of resilience required to perform well in the medical profession.

Conversation – Accountability

Mikey was disappointed in himself. He had let his research project slide. It had been nearly six months since he had discussed it with Sam. They were looking at local data on venous thromboembolism in pregnancy, and seeing whether or not thrombophilia testing had been done appropriately. At the time he was enthusiastic about it – it would be publishable data and he would be first author. But the enthusiasm soon gave way to boredom, which meant that it got pushed down the priority list; well behind work, study and Netflix (though not necessarily in that order).

There were a few problems. Ethics submissions were painfully detailed. Data collection was like watching paint dry. Reviewing the literature was frustrating, because there didn't seem to be a clear consensus on what 'appropriate' testing was. So instead of working through the issues, he had just let it slide. Put it on the backburner. On a very low heat.

Still, although he was disappointed in himself, he was more worried about disappointing Sam. They had a meeting in five minutes, and he had to tell Sam that since their last meeting he had done precisely nothing on the project.

He walked down the corridor to Sam's office, which was a familiar walk by now. They had met about once a month, sometimes formally, other times informally. He always seemed to walk away feeling better about things after a conversation with Sam – like his problem had a solution, or at the very least like he had an idea about what the next step was. He had usually held up his side of the bargain, but this time was different.

He reached the office. As per usual, Sam's door was open. Sam heard Mikey approach, looked up, and smiled.

'Mikey, come in,' he said.

'Hi, Sam. How's it going?' asked Mikey.

'Going well. How about you?' asked Sam.

'I'm okay. Busy, as per usual.'

'Aren't we all?' Sam sympathised.

Mikey took a seat.

'Okay, I've got in my diary that we're talking about the VTE project today. How's it coming along?' asked Sam.

Mikey exhaled audibly. 'Frankly, not good. I've been busy. I haven't really looked at it for a few months. I'm sorry.'

'That's okay. You don't have to apologise, Mikey. Research isn't easy. Remember this is your goal, and your paper. What's been the problem? Loss of enthusiasm?'

'Big time. How'd you know?'

Sam chuckled. 'I wasn't born yesterday. You forget that I was where you are not that long ago. You mentioned you are feeling busy – are you too busy?'

'Maybe. I don't think so. I'm a bit stressed, but coping. The timetable we made at the start of the year is helpful to keep track of things.'

'That's good; some people need a little bit of stress to be effective. But we need to be careful of burnout. Are you getting any down time?'

'Yeah, I've got a couple of weeks off coming up. Heading home to see the folks. Should be refreshing.'

'Good,' said Sam. 'Try and spend that time relaxing. Don't think about work. Exams are still months away, and the project can wait. Make sure you get some down time.'

'That's the plan,' said Mikey. 'Mum and Dad won't let me do any work!'

'Good. Now, let's talk about the matter at hand. Why do you think you've lost enthusiasm?'

'I don't know. Maybe research just isn't for me. Data collection is painful. Family history isn't always documented. Sometimes testing has been done at a private lab which is difficult to access. I'm just starting to see what a huge job it is to get reliable data,' lamented Mikey.

'Welcome to research!' said Sam, with mock enthusiasm. 'It can be like pulling teeth. Look, Mikey, this feeling is universal. Go and talk to a PhD student and ask them. Frustration with data collection is natural. Don't feel like a failure because you've stalled. But just remember, some people are well suited to research, and others aren't. It's okay if research isn't your thing.'

'That's good to hear, and a bit of a weight off to be honest. I can't imagine doing this for the rest of my life,' said Mikey.

'Well, that's fantastic!' exclaimed Sam.

'Wait, what? How is this fantastic?' Mikey asked, a confused look furrowing his brow.

'Mikey, the whole point of this mentoring exercise is to help you develop into the kind of doctor you want to be. Part of that process is figuring out what kind of doctor you don't want to be. And you've figured out that you probably don't want to be a researcher. That helps us set goals,' Sam explained.

'So you're saying I don't have to do any research?' Mikey asked hopefully.

Sam chuckled again. 'Careful. There's a difference between being a researcher and doing some research. Research is part of your curriculum, same as learning how to read an ECG and manage pneumonia. Why do you think that is?'

'Because punishment is character building?' Mikey joked.

Sam laughed. 'You really don't like research do you?'

'No, not really,' said Mikey. 'But I suppose I can see some advantages. It will look good on my CV to have something published. It will also help me to get a job in future.'

'Yes, those things are important. But that's not the only reason. Doing your own research gives you an appreciation for the utility and limitations of doing research. This retrospective audit you're doing – all of your problems with data collection? This is why retrospective data is inherently flawed and needs to be interpreted with caution. The data isn't easy to extract. It's open to all kind of bias, and it's not controlled. You also get a much better handle on statistics, and how to read and interpret the papers that will be relevant to your practice in the future. You develop a much greater understanding of these things by doing some research of your own,' Sam explained.

'I guess you're right,' said Mikey. 'I never saw it that way.'

'That's okay, that's what I'm here for. Now, all of that being said, we're not so far into this that you can't stop if you want to. If you don't think you want to do this project, that's okay. We can review your goals, and focus on other things.'

Mikey thought about it for a minute. Deep down he knew the project was a good one, and that it was good for him.

'Sam, you're right. This is good for me. I'm going to do it. Can you stay on me about it?' asked Mikey?

'I'll do better than that,' said Sam. 'Last week the medical school was onto us asking if we had any projects that some enthusiastic medical students might be able to chip in with. I think we should make contact and see if one of them would like to help out with the data collection. What do you think?'

'That's a fantastic idea. That would really help take the pressure off,' said Mikey.

'Great,' said Sam. 'I think you've made the right decision here. Who knows – you might even grow to love it!'

'If only your enthusiasm were infectious. Thanks, Sam.'

'My pleasure, Mikey.'

Scenario precis

Mentoring isn't easy. If it were, you wouldn't be reading this book. Mentoring can be disappointing, especially when the mentee does not develop or perform in the way you had planned.

Mikey is a good mentee – he's enthusiastic, hardworking, generally competent and learns quickly. If even 'good' mentees drop the ball sometimes, it is not surprising that others can really struggle. This is where using Evaluation (Tool #9) is useful, to explore what happened and what resulted, particularly when there is a mismatch between the desired outcome and the actual outcome.

In this scenario, Mikey suffers the familiar struggle of data collection fatigue. He and Sam have to decide whether or not the goal of publishing a paper remains a realistic goal. After checking on Mikey's well-being using Resilience work (Tool #6), Sam probes to see if the goal truly is realistic and whether Mikey wants to continue. He then offers assistance in the form of engaging a medical student to start collecting data, to help make the goal more achievable. Without Evaluation (Tool #9) and adjustment to the plan for goal achievement, Mikey's research goal may have fallen by the wayside. In this case, Mikey chose to continue pursuing his goal. However, it is important to remember that goals are for the mentee's benefit, and may be reviewed and changed if they cease to be relevant to the mentee.

Conversation – Understanding and addressing performance problems that are complex

Mikey stood in line for coffee just before clinic. He was in a foul mood. Study group had gone longer than it needed to last night, and he slept late. Out of their study group of three, one of them was not pulling his weight. His name was Tom, and he was beginning to make Mikey frustrated and angry.

Last night he showed up to study group at the third member's house, Rebecca, or 'Bec' as she preferred. He came late. Mumbled an apology about being busy, then proceeded to tell them that he hadn't looked over his share of the study material or prepared anything.

This wasn't the first time. It was a recurring pattern over the last few weeks. Tom seemed keen at the start, but it seemed like he was getting lazy. Mikey knew he himself had a lot of flaws, but he took pride in working hard, particularly when it came to his responsibilities with his colleagues. He had hoped that his efforts would have been reciprocated by his colleagues.

He could tell Bec was getting frustrated too. She was more patient than Mikey, but Tom's laziness was even getting to her. They had discussed it briefly last night after Tom had left, and had decided to confront Tom about it at their next meeting, give him an ultimatum. Pull your weight, or do it on your own.

He must had been scowling, because at that moment Sam walked by and said 'Come on Mikey, the coffee here isn't that bad!'

Mikey was jolted out of his brooding and forced a smile. 'Yeah, it's okay I guess. You want one?'

'Sure, thanks.'

The line moved and Mikey was next at the counter. He ordered and sat down at one of the tables next to Sam to wait. Busy morning. Might be a few minutes.

'So Mikey, how's it going?' asked Sam.

Mikey thought about telling Sam about Tom, but then thought better of it. He didn't want to make Sam think less of Tom.

'It's okay. Just tired. Busy, exams in only a couple of months. Feeling the pinch, I guess.'

'Fair enough, we've all been there. Coping alright?' asked Sam sympathetically.

'Yeah, I think so. Just have to put in the hard yards for the next two months then it's all over!'

'How is study coming along?' enquired Sam.

Mikey hesitated. 'Could be better.'

'How so?' asked Sam.

Mikey hesitated again. Sam had this way of asking the right questions.

'Mikey – just remember everything we discuss is confidential. You don't have to talk if you don't want to, but I can see something's bothering you. I can't help unless you tell me.'

'Well, it's not really anything to do with me. I'm fine. It's about one of my colleagues,' Mikey said reluctantly.

'Confidentiality still applies. I can be impartial. Learning how to deal with difficulties with colleagues is part of any professional development,' offered Sam.

Mikey exhaled. Sam was right. Brooding over the situation like a child wasn't helping. He needed to find a professional way to deal with this. 'Well, it's a problem with study group. One of our members isn't pulling his weight, and it's really starting to get to me and to the other member. We're working our butts off, and he's coasting, using our notes. It's frustrating, because now the work is essentially divided between two instead of three, which wasn't the deal at the start. It's not really fair – we're planning to give him an ultimatum.'

'That's rough,' agreed Sam. 'Especially so close to the exam. Why do you think this person isn't pulling their weight?'

'I don't know, laziness I guess,' replied Mikey, realising that he'd never actually asked the question why.

'It's worth thinking about. You're stressed, understandably. Everyone is at this stage. Try not to let that cloud your judgment. Think about your colleague. Has he given any signs that there's more to this than laziness?'

'Well, I didn't think he was lazy at the start. That's why we asked him to join the group. Lately though, he's been...distant. Not really engaging.' Suddenly it dawned on Mikey. 'Oh no. He's depressed, isn't he? Wow. I feel like a jerk.'

'It's a concern,' said Sam. 'He may just be too stressed to be functional. Either way, sounds like he might need a friend first, before an ultimatum.'

'I can't believe I missed it. I mean, I'm no psychiatrist but this is psych 101. What should I do?'

'Identifying the problem goes halfway to solving it. I suggest you– '

Sam was cut off by a shrill, loud voice calling 'Two takeaway lattes for Mikey; coffee for Mikey!'

'Hold that thought,' Mikey said, and pushed his chair back and walked to the counter to get the coffees. He brought them back and sat down. 'You were saying?'

'I suggest you just have a chat to him. Give him the benefit of the doubt. Demeanor is important. Let him know that the study is secondary. First priority is that he's okay. If you think it's serious, and you're out of your depth – encourage him to see his GP, or get him plugged into the hospital counselling service. We have to look after our colleagues.'

'You're right. You're totally right. It really wasn't fair of me to go on the offensive straight away. That would have made it worse,' said Mikey.

'Possibly. Now, it's still important to make sure that your study is on track. How's it going?' asked Sam, taking the first sip of coffee.

'We should be okay. We did what you suggested, and structured in a contingency. We have two unstructured weeks in the study schedule that we can dip into to try and catch up what we've missed. I'm glad we did that!'

'Something similar happened to me the month before my fellowship exams. My wife got appendicitis and had to spend five days in hospital. Since then I've told everyone who asks to give themselves a bit of extra time,' said Sam.

'It's good advice. Thanks, Sam, as always.'

'As always, it's my pleasure.'

Scenario precis

This scenario is complex, in the sense that factors outside of Mikey's control are having an effect on his progress. It is also complex in the sense that it encompasses both personal and professional aspects, and deals with sensitive information. In addition to Purposeful communication (Tool #1), two tools being displayed here are Resilience work (Tool #6) and Confidentiality (Tool #8).

Sam's posture towards his junior staff is one of care and dedication; this is one reason why he is able to identify issues of well-being so readily. However, it is also something that he tries to instill in his mentee, with the hope and expectation that Mikey will one day be able to do the same for others.

This scenario also helps to highlight the importance of Confidentiality (Tool #8). Without being confident that the communication was confidential, Mikey would not have shared his concerns, and the situation could have deteriorated. This was particularly true, as Sam was Tom's consultant, and Mikey did not want Sam to think less of Tom, for fear that it might reflect badly on him within the unit.

Dealing with sensitive information like this requires considerable communication skills and objectivity.

Conversation – Improving performance of an essential task

Mikey was waiting in Sam's office for Sam, who was running late after clinic. It was one of their regular meetings where they discussed Mikey's goals. It had been six months since Mikey went to Sam with his lack of confidence with performing a lumbar puncture. Since then, Mikey had logged nearly twenty successful procedures, and was starting to feel confident, and was beginning to teach his residents and interns.

Then came his 'back down to Earth' moment. He recently had a patient, a young woman with visual disturbances and headache, and he suspected idiopathic intracranial hypertension, which required a lumbar puncture for diagnosis. She was obese and had difficulty getting into the correct position due to chronic back pain. This combination of factors made the procedure very difficult, and Mikey had not been able to complete it. Eventually the patient had the procedure done in Radiology the following day.

Mikey was frustrated with himself, so when Sam arrived Mikey thought it might be worthwhile seeing if he had any more advice.

'Mikey, sorry I'm late,' said Sam as he came in and sat down across from Mikey.

'No problem at all. Clinic can be a nightmare,' Mikey sympathized.

'It was a busy one. How are you doing?' asked Sam.

'Not too bad,' said Mikey. 'I was hoping we could chat more about lumbar punctures.' 'Sure thing,' replied Sam. 'You told me they were going well. What's up?'

'Well, they were going well. I had one last week that I couldn't get no matter what.' Mikey explained the scenario to Sam, who nodded in understanding.

'This is common,' said Sam. 'Competency isn't an on-off switch. There are varying levels of competency. Certainly you sound competent enough for your training purposes, but I suppose now it becomes a question of how 'expert' do you want to become?'

'I quite like the procedure, and I'm thinking about neurology as a specialty, so I'd like to be able to do it well,' said Mikey. 'Also, it's a pain in the neck to have to organise it through Radiology. It would be much simpler if I could just do it.'

'Fair enough,' replied Sam. 'Expertise is on the same spectrum as competence, it's just that an expert is able to perform the task at a higher level of performance and in a wider range of circumstances. A junior surgical registrar might be able to take out an appendix if it's uncomplicated, but you might need an expert for a ruptured appendix with prior surgery and lots of adhesions.'

'Right – so other than more practice, how do I develop expertise?'

'Well, practice is clearly the most important thing. But there are a few ways you can capitalise on your practice. First, think about what went wrong in this case. Analyse it critically. Was the position wrong? Was your angle wrong? Were your landmarks off? Next time, correct these aspects of your performance. Then, seek out the difficult cases. The ones that nobody wants to do. Critically analyse your performance again. Don't beat yourself up for missing the difficult ones; treat it as a learning exercise. What went right? What went wrong? Talk to people who are already experts and get some of their tips – sometimes the smallest things make a difference!'

'Good point. I might try and catch up with Dr. Costello. I know he's really good at them and gave me some hints when I was getting started. I'll see if he has any other tips. Thanks, Sam.'

'My pleasure, Mikey.'

Scenario precis

Whilst a doctor may be competent to perform a procedure in a controlled environment, they may not be sufficiently competent to do so if there are complicating factors. Such is the case here with Mikey. Anatomical variation and patient factors made a procedure he was familiar with and competent at far more difficult to the point where he could not complete it. A higher level of expertise was required to be able to complete the task.

Improving performance is often viewed as something that occurs passively, which is true to a point. Deliberate practice, particularly with a more experienced operator using Goal-directed interaction (Tool #3), can improve performance faster and further.

In this scenario, Mikey starts to recognise his own developmental needs, needing Sam only to guide. The role of mentor becomes more 'hands-off' when it comes to improving performance where there is already competency.

Conversation – Work-life balance

Mikey was rushing out the door of the hospital at 7:30pm, eating a sandwich that was supposed to be lunch but had become dinner after a twelve-hour non-stop day. Now he was heading home to get some more study done before getting up tomorrow and doing it all again. As he walked along towards his car, he saw Sam in the parking lot about to get into his car and head home.

'Have a good night, Sam!' Mikey said as he approached.

'Mikey, what are you still doing here so late?' asked Sam.

'Busy day. Three MET calls, seven admissions and a resident off sick. What's your excuse?'

'Had a teleconference that ran late. You've been late out for the last few weeks, I've noticed,' said Sam, with a hint of concern in his voice.

'Yeah, it's been busy. There are new residents on the team, they are still finding their feet.'

'Are you managing to keep up with study?' asked Sam.

'Keeping to schedule for the moment!' said Mikey.

'Right – when was the last time you had a break? Did something fun?' asked Sam.

'Fun? What's that?' asked Mikey, only half joking.

'Seriously, Mikey, you'll burn out if you keep pushing yourself this hard. When's the last time you cycled?' Sam probed.

Mikey thought for a while. 'It's got a few cobwebs,' he said.

'Take a look at your schedule. See where you can fit an hour or two per week for a bit of down time. You'll probably find that your study improves. Your mood and energy certainly will,' Sam offered.

Mikey thought for a moment. He knew Sam was right. He couldn't run on adrenaline forever.

'You're right, as usual,' said Mikey. 'I think I'll ride this weekend. Try to make it regular. Thanks Sam.'

'Good, now get out of here! The hospital will still be here tomorrow!' said Sam, as he climbed into his car.

Scenario precis

Work-life balance is something many doctors struggle with. This is an understandable, if not unavoidable part of many medical careers. Diseases don't read textbooks, nor do they respect social hours and public holidays. Add to that a rigorous post-graduate training schedule, and the things outside of work that one enjoys can quickly fall lower and lower on the priority list.

In this scenario, Sam uses Resilience work (Tool #6) as well as Career guidance (Tool #7) in order to raise Mikey's awareness that his work habits have begun to have a detrimental effect on his life. Many readers would be familiar with this, with some pockets of the profession maintaining a culture that life is medicine.

Sam helps Mikey to see that a healthy life outside of work not only improves his well-being, but will likely make him a better doctor in the future.

Felt separation

Conversation – Concluding mentoring

It had been a long two years. Mikey was not the doctor he was when he started here. He had come a long way. His time here was coming to an end; he was moving on to the next phase of his training at a larger center. He was moving in one week.

He would remember this place fondly. He thought back to when he started; fresh-faced, and basically scared out of his mind that he would now be the one making decisions. He remembered being mortally afraid of doing what he now considered second nature. Things like running a code, or managing a seizure. He silently marveled at how amazing the human brain and body was, so adaptable to new skills, environments and challenges.

One of those challenges had been his exams. He thought he would really struggle with them. He was a practical person, good with his hands, but in the past he had just done enough to get by at medical school. Middle of the class. Nothing special.

How things change. He had found a specialty he was passionate about, and a mentor who had helped him to apply his strengths, and all of a sudden study became relevant. Helpful. Perhaps even, enjoyable? Well, maybe not that far. Either way, he passed the exams. He passed them well. They were difficult, to be sure. Still scary. But not scary like meeting a lion in the wild. More like meeting a lion in a zoo, tame and relatively safe. To be respected, certainly. To have a healthy fear of, sure. But in fear of your life? That seemed to be how some of his colleagues saw the exam. They were so very stressed, as though life would be over if they failed. Mikey used to see it that way, but as the exam came closer he realised something. He had worked hard; he knew the content. So he walked in there, sat down, and wrote the exam. And passed. Well. Very well, in fact.

A wry smile came across his face. He let his mind drift to the other things he'd learned since he'd been here, and the people he'd met. He let the nostalgia wash over him. He had become fond of this place; truth be told he didn't really want to leave, but he knew it was for the best. His new position was in a tertiary center, fast paced and full of experiences.

He thought of Sam. Mikey was very grateful to him. He always seemed to have time, and seemingly infinite patience, despite a busy schedule. He had a real knack not just for teaching, but for developing people.

Mikey looked down at the bottle in his hands. It was an 18 year Glen Livet, a single malt scotch whisky from Scotland and one of Sam's favorites. He had bought it for him as a thank you gift, but it felt entirely inadequate. It was a token only. Still, better than nothing, he thought.

He walked down the now very familiar corridor to Sam's office. It was late afternoon on a Friday, and work was winding up for the week. Sam had wanted to catch up one last time before Mikey left, and late on a Friday was a good time, because nobody in their right mind had a clinic late on a Friday afternoon.

He approached the office. The door was open, as usual. Sam was sitting at his desk, neatly stacked charts and paperwork on his desk, as usual. Sam looked up as he heard Mikey at the door and smiled, as usual. More nostalgia.

'Mikey,' said Sam, 'Come in and sit down.'

'Thanks,' replied Mikey, and took Sam's offer and sat across the desk from him.
'Your last week next week, how are you feeling?' Sam asked.

'I'm okay. Truth be told I'm a bit nostalgic about it all. It's been a great two years.'

'It sure has. You've come a long way,' said Sam.

'You're right about that. And you're a big part of why, Sam. So before I get too nostalgic, I want to say thanks. Sincerely. You've been great. Here's a bottle of your favorite as a token of my gratitude. I know it's not much, but –'

'Is that the 18 year!?' exclaimed Sam, reaching over eagerly to take the bottle. 'Wow. This is great stuff. You really didn't have to, so thanks.'

Mikey chuckled. 'It's the least I could do. You've gone above and beyond to help me these last two years.'

'Well,' said Sam, 'I appreciate that you think so. But I really don't see it that way. Developing the next generation is really part of our job. Besides, I enjoy it. It's not every day you get to make a difference in someone's life.'

'Except, you know, if you're a doctor and you save lives every day,' Mikey joked.

'Touché,' Sam chuckled. 'Seriously though, you have come a long way here. Do you remember what we set out to do two years ago? What your goals were?'

'Yeah, of course. Pass exams, publish a paper, and learn how to be competent day to day.'

'How do you think we went?' probed Sam.

'Well, I got through the exams; they turned out to have less teeth than I thought they would.'

'Most people who are well prepared feel that way,' said Sam.

'We did finally get that damned paper published too. That medical student you sent me – Shu-en – she was a machine. I don't understand how someone can be so enthusiastic about activated protein C resistance.'

'Some people have the gift of enjoying research,' said Sam. 'Have you come around to it?'

Mikey made a face. 'I will admit, it's nice to have something published with your name on the front page. But I highly doubt I'll make a career out of it,' he said.

'That's ok. Knowing what you don't want to do is as important as knowing what you want to do,' Sam replied. 'What about the third goal – becoming comfortable and competent in your day to day work. How are you going in that space?'

'Pretty well, I think. I mean don't get me wrong, there are certainly times where I still need help, but I'm comfortable with the majority of things now.'

'I would agree. I've seen you on the wards, and in the clinic. Your procedural skills are excellent and improving all the time. Your clinical judgment is really quite mature, and continuing to develop. I'm very happy with your progress,' said Sam.

'That's good to know!'

'Is there anything you wanted to achieve that you haven't been able to?' asked Sam.

Mikey thought for a moment. 'I think work-life balance is still a struggle. Knowing I was likely only going to be here for two years from the start, I thought it was better to throw myself into work and try make the most of it. But now I kind of regret that, a little. My social life hasn't exactly been vibrant!'

'It's a hard balance,' Sam conceded. 'Just remember, these things are for a time. Exams are a non-negotiable, they do eat into your social time. It's a fact of life. But what happens now is up to you. Some people will continue to throw themselves into work, because they love it, at the expense of their social life. Other people will pull back on work for family, friends. The only person who knows the right thing to do is you – just make sure it's a positive decision, one way or the other. I'd hate for you to get ten years down the track and realise that all you've done is work, and haven't taken the time to do the other things you wanted. Work will always be there. It will always demand more of your time if you allow it. If you want it not to, you have to make a positive decision for it not to.'

Mikey nodded, contemplative. 'One last lesson, huh Sam?' he asked with a wry smile.

'I guess so,' said Sam. 'Actually, Mikey, I have a favour to ask of you.'

'Sure,' replied Mikey, 'Anything. What do you need?'

'This mentoring we've been doing. What you've learned. In a couple of weeks when you start at your new job, I want you to find someone your junior who you can help out in a similar way.'

'You mean, like, pay it forward?' asked Mikey.

'Something like that,' said Sam. 'If we want our profession to continue to improve and grow and evolve, we need to invest in the juniors who are coming through. Find a mentor, and find someone to mentor.'

'Fair enough,' said Mikey. 'I still don't really feel like I'm senior enough to teach anyone else anything. I'm not sure I could do it very well, but I will give it a try.'

'You'll surprise yourself,' said Sam. 'You now know what it takes to produce change, to intentionally help someone develop. All you need to do is help someone apply that framework to their personal circumstances.'

'Fair enough. I'll give it a go. I might be calling you for advice though!'

'You're most welcome to. Now, it's after five o'clock. Work is finished. I've got two glasses in the cabinet – what would you say to a celebratory nip?' asked Sam.

'I thought you'd never ask,' replied Mikey.

Scenario precis

With this final scenario, the mentoring partnership between Mikey and Sam is formally concluded. Sam guides Mikey in evaluating the two-year mentoring partnership and process using Evaluation (Tool #9) and also in felt separation, from Partnership (Tool #2).

It is important for a final mentoring conversation to include a review of the successes and failures of the partnership. Mikey and Sam review their original goals, and thankfully find more wins than losses. Acknowledging difficulties is equally important, as this gives the mentor an opportunity to learn from experience, and gives the mentee some new goals for their next mentoring partnership.

In this case, Mikey is moving away, so there is closure. However, many mentoring partnerships will face a more open-ended conclusion. Ideally, the anticipated duration of mentoring is discussed at the beginning, as it helps with timely progress towards the defined goals. If a partnership has achieved all that you wish it to achieve by the end of the defined period, the partnership has two options. New goals can be set and the partnership can continue. Alternatively, the partnership can be concluded. The mentee may wish to form another mentoring partnership. Just as it is useful for trainees to experience multiple different hospitals and healthcare settings, so it is useful for them to work with different mentors.

17. The versatile mentor

Toolkit variations

In this book, we have deconstructed mentoring to a partnership and process for development. The partnership requires relational work, and the process requires developmental work. The ten tools of the intentional mentor can be used to accomplish the mentor's part of this work and you will find uses for the intentional mentor's toolkit in diverse mentoring scenarios. In practice, the elements of mentoring do not have such neat divisions, and diverse mentoring scenarios will challenge you to combine elements fluidly and in novel ways for particular purposes. A number of mentee-related factors will affect how you might use your tools. Mentee-related factors include:

- seniority
- specialty
- participation in a mentoring program
- transition points
- the number of mentees requesting your assistance
- whether they are your supervisee.

The senior mentee

As the seniority of the mentee increases, higher-level skills may appear in their job description. The more senior the mentee, the more likely they are to be involved in supervision and management. Knowing the mentee's job description will help you to help the mentee who is in a more senior position. Examples of mentoring priorities by postgraduate year are illustrated in Table 15. It is important to note that these will vary depending on context, for example, the early streaming to specialty training that happens in some locations, or the additional performance requirements associated with practice in rural settings.

Table 15. Typical mentoring priorities by postgraduate year

POSTGRADUATE YEAR	COMMON DEVELOPMENTAL PRIORITIES
1	Consolidate learning Apply knowledge from medical school
2	Decide on career path Broaden experience of rural and regional settings Continue to learn and apply learning
3-5 (early vocational training)	Apply for a training program Acquire training-specific competencies Prepare and undertake exams
6-8 (late vocational training)	Consolidate learning Learn consultant-level decision making Conduct research
9-10+ (consultant)	Become comfortable with high-level clinical decision making Learn how to manage staff and junior doctors Plan career development

The mentee in a vocational training program

To be most helpful to the mentee in a vocational training program, you will need to be familiar with the distinct requirements and curriculum and performance standards of the speciality. These tend to get more and more specific naturally because they pertain to a specialty. Educational supervisors are in a unique position to be involved in mentoring, above and beyond their assigned educational supervisor roles. Ideally, assigned educational supervisors who are not line managers will act as mentors to their trainees, though at times this will not be possible. (In Chapter 6, p.75 we mentioned the conflict of interest that can arise when the mentor is required to also be the formal assessor). If you are in a different field to the mentee, do not assume you have nothing to offer as a mentor. Provided you are familiar with the curriculum and performance standards, you can be of assistance, often in very helpful ways.

The mentee in a mentoring program

'Formal' and 'informal' are descriptors applied to mentoring to classify the level of organisational involvement in mentoring. *Informal mentoring* is mentoring that occurs without the assistance of the organisation in supporting the partnership. An example of informal mentoring is mentoring that occurs between a senior doctor and a junior doctor who agree to collaborate on the junior doctor's development. *Formal mentoring* is mentoring that occurs with the assistance of an organisation in supporting the partnership. An example of formal mentoring is the mentoring that occurs through a mentoring program. Mentors who are involved in formal mentoring may be required to adjust their use of the tools in ways that are specified by the organisation. There may be a requirement to engage with the program coordinator as well as the mentee, provide evaluation data, and focus on particular developmental outcomes. The mentee should be informed of any requirements or conditions of mentoring set by a third party prior to participating in mentoring.

The mentee in transition

Certain times of the year are associated with greater demand for mentoring. This is especially relevant at times of transition, for example, at the start of the year when the mentee is progressing to a higher level of seniority. At mid-year, demand for mentoring can also be high coinciding with doctors seeking guidance in relation to applying for jobs and training programs. Towards the end of the year, the mentee may wish to discuss outcomes of job applications, come to terms with what those scenarios mean for them, and explore options. Resilience work may have greater relevance to the mentee at times of transition.

The volume of mentees

Time management will be particularly important if you are working with numerous mentees. How many mentees can you assist, showing CARE? It is better to do an excellent job with fewer mentees than a mediocre job with many mentees. If the need for mentoring is great, consider group mentoring on occasions, and encourage your colleagues to share the workload and get involved in mentoring.

The supervisor who acts as a mentor

We consider supervisors who provide junior medical colleagues with individually relevant support, challenge and facilitation, to be supervisors who act as mentors. The intentional mentor's toolkit has utility to supervisors who act as mentors, however some variations in the use of the toolkit will apply. For example, confidentiality is less defined; if the supervisee does not meet competency and performance standards the supervisor may be required to involve others in remediating the supervisee. Goal-directed interactions will have more focused end-points that are dictated by the curriculum and established learning objectives.

Overall, mentoring is more likely to focus on developing the supervisee's performance in their current work setting. However, the supervisor who acts as a mentor goes one step further than what would otherwise be expected of their role. They engage with the supervisee on a level beyond ensuring that the supervisee meets the minimum required curriculum and performance standards in the specialty. They endeavour to help the supervisee to realise their aspirational state of development. The focus of mentoring extends beyond the supervisee's attainment of competence and acceptable performance, to attainment of peak performance and resilience.

One of the convenient features of being a supervisor who acts as a mentor is that the structure for relational and developmental work is largely in place already. It is advisable to discuss with the supervisee at the start of the supervising period whether or not they would be interested in a mentoring partnership. If they are interested, the starting point is to form an agreement and set goals that go beyond those of a supervisory relationship. Ensure that the supervisee does not feel pressured into agreeing, as they may already be involved in one or more mentoring partnerships that meet their needs.

18. Developing a culture of mentoring in medicine

Collaborating for change

> Imagine a teaching hospital where the sharing of knowledge and expertise is the cultural norm and readily given, where collaboration rather than competition is the driving force of progress, where conversations are constructive and lead to learning, insight and effective action, where a culture of care permeates the work environment, and patients do well as a result. How good would that be? This is not just wishful thinking; it is a real possibility for the future through mentoring.
> (Salvador & Collings, 2014, p. 24)

The ultimate purpose of mentoring doctors is to change medical practice in ways that improve health outcomes of patients. A culture of mentoring, driven by diverse contributors, enables this on a large scale. Doctors, health service leaders, health policy makers, colleges, regulatory bodies and oversight committees, advocacy groups and education agencies can all contribute to developing a culture of mentoring in medicine.

Doctors participate in mentoring as mentors and mentees

A culture of mentoring begins with individual doctors valuing their own and their colleagues' development as doctors, and choosing to have a positive influence on colleagues. Most of us are aware of how much of an influence our senior doctors had on us. Most have had at least a few great experiences, where we were inspired to learn, to develop, to grow. Most have also had difficult experiences, where we felt belittled, intimidated or bullied. Nobody ever says "I want to be like the doctor who belittled me." You will seldom meet a junior doctor or medical student who one day dreams of scaring his or her trainees into submission. The almost universal experience of junior doctors, when they have such encounters, is to say "I'll never be like that! When I'm a senior doctor, I'll remember what it's like to be junior, and I'll be kind to people."

Think back on your medical training thus far. Who inspired you? Were they intelligent? Probably. Were they competent? Almost certainly. However, it is a good bet that they were more than that. They were inspiring. They took an interest in you. They wanted you to develop.

To change medical culture, we need to make positive role modeling the norm. We need to be the kind of doctors who inspire our junior medical colleagues, so that they mature into the kind of doctors who inspire their junior medical colleagues.

Leaders endorse mentoring and promote collegiality

To change culture, change at the individual level is not enough. We must change our units, our departments, our hospitals. The groundswell of enthusiastic junior doctors and mentors must be supported by endorsement and facilitation from the existing leadership structures.

Endorsement of mentoring from leaders makes it acceptable for doctors to care not only for patients but also for each other. Endorsement may take many forms, for example, granting permission for mentoring to take place through mentoring programs, and permitting mentors and mentees to have mentoring conversations in work time. Providing spaces conducive to conversation, such as meeting rooms or doctors' lounges, can be a visible indicator of endorsement of mentoring partnerships and collegiality. Leaders can also actively engage in and model mentoring participation.

Policy makers enable mentoring

Policy makers within local, state and national agencies enable mentoring to occur when they formulate policy that prioritises mentoring as a strategy for doctor development. Policy may enable mentoring to occur on a particular scale (e.g. at a local health service, state or national level), at a particular volume, with a particular focus, or for particular target groups of doctors. Policy may relate to making mentor training accessible, targeting achievement of specific outcomes such as resilience, providing dedicated time for mentoring, offering incentives for participating in mentoring, and funding a mentoring program for a community of doctors, and more.

Colleges resource mentoring partnerships

Colleges perform a vital role in producing high quality resources, including curriculum and performance standards documents, that guide mentors in their work with mentees. Additionally, most colleges facilitate partnerships between trainees and at least one supervisor who ensures that the trainee is meeting his or her training requirements. Elements of mentoring exist in these supervisor-trainee partnerships, and this existing structure is fertile ground for supervisors to act as mentors.

Regulatory bodies and oversight committees promote mentoring

Regulatory bodies, such as registration and accreditation authorities, are in a position to promote mentoring as a strategy for doctor development. Methods may include monitoring compliance with policies and standards, recognising and encouraging organisational support for mentoring, and mandating peer consultation. In the psychology profession in Australia, peer consultation is a requirement of the continuing professional development registration standard. This could serve as a precedent for the medical profession. Practically speaking, local training hubs and committees are well placed to promote mentoring, give oversight to mentoring initiatives and provide structure, support and governance to mentoring programs.

Advocacy groups address systemic problems

Agencies providing advocacy, such as Australian Medical Association, can identify and raise awareness of systemic problems affecting doctors in practice. They may also conduct research and generate findings in relation to doctors' normative, comparative and expressed needs. With this information, mentors can tailor comprehensive support, challenge and facilitation, specific to individual needs.

Education agencies coordinate programs

Medical education units at teaching hospitals, and other training providers, can contribute administrative support for mentoring initiatives and programs. Administrative support may include matching mentors and mentees, training mentors, hosting events, assisting with program activities, maintaining the program's profile, and evaluating the program.

Figure 21 shows the mentoring collaborations that can ultimately lead to widespread change in medical practice in ways that improve health outcomes of patients.

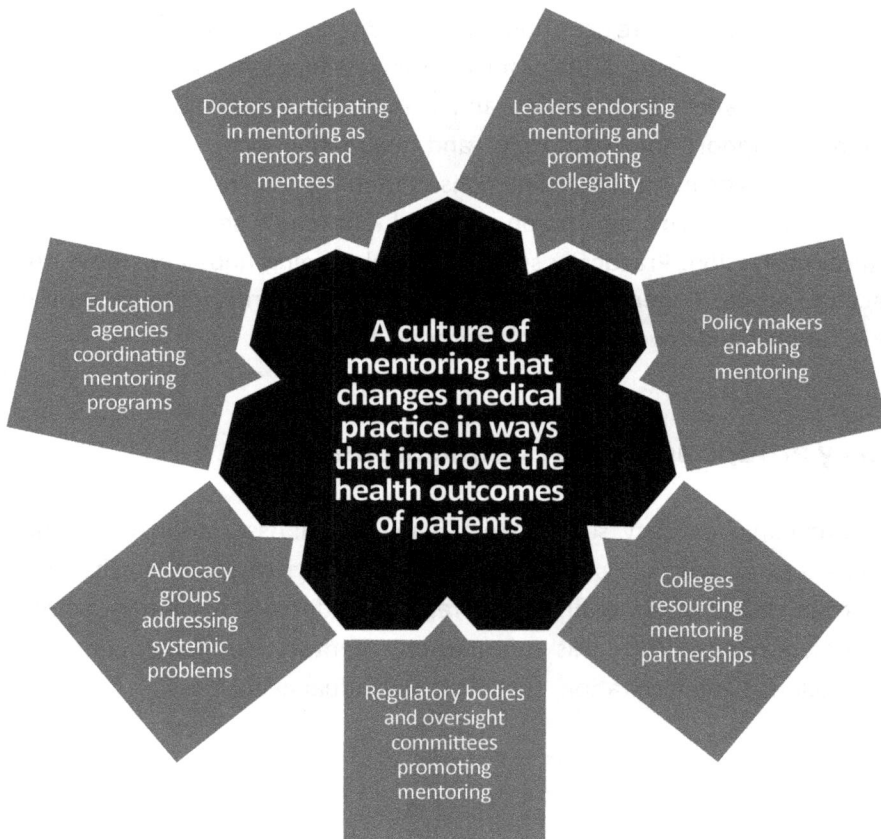

Figure 21. Through mentoring, changing medical practice in ways that improve health outcomes of patients

Appendices

Appendices

Appendix A
The science of developing performance

"The field of medicine — as is the case with most other professional fields — lacks a strong tradition of supporting the training and further improvement of practicing professionals. It is assumed that medical professionals are able to figure out, on their own, effective practice techniques and apply them to improve their performance. In short, the implicit assumption in medical training has been that if you provide doctors with the necessary knowledge — in medical school, through medical journals, or through seminars and continuing medical education classes — this should be sufficient."
(Ericsson, 2016)

This section focuses on the theory of developing performance, and in particular, skill development. It includes practical guidelines for fostering the mentee's skill development using Ericsson's principles of deliberate practice.

Acquisition and improvement of mediating mechanisms

After the mentee achieves a functional level of performance of a skill, increasing experience and time in a field using the skill does not necessarily generate further improvements in performance. Developing performance of a particular skill occurs through acquiring and improving mediating mechanisms. Mediating mechanisms are the processes of the brain and body that produce and control the performance, and also provide the mechanisms that can be altered for improved performance with practice (Lehmann & Gruber, 2006).

Improvement of a skill can be described as passing through one state of development to the next, as shown in Figure A1. On the x-axis are states of development, consisting of mediating mechanisms. On the y-axis are levels of performance. Each level of performance is produced by acquiring and improving the mechanisms that mediate execution of the skill (Ericsson, 2006).

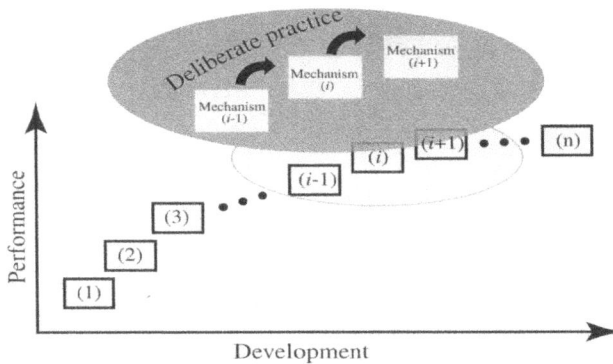

Figure A1. Developing performance
Source: Ericsson et al. (2006)

Mediating mechanisms are specific to each task within task performance conditions. Ability-related mediating mechanisms may be classified broadly as cognitive and physiological mediating mechanisms. Typical cognitive mediating mechanisms include attention, perception, knowledge stored as procedural and declarative memory, and retrieval structures for long-term memory. Physiological mediating mechanisms include muscle movement patterns, posture, force, torque and energy. These cognitive and physiological mediating mechanisms create the potential for performance. Trait-related and other mediating mechanisms contribute to actual performance. In doctors, notable trait-related mediating mechanisms include motivation, drive, will, self-efficacy and curiosity. Jones (2014) chooses curiosity as the greatest of the traits related to excellent care quality. She explains that a physician with a curious mind does not necessarily know all the answers, and may not be the 'smartest' graduate of medical school, but is a great detective, and does not rest until problems are solved. Given that doctors require endurance and stamina to perform, resilience may also be considered a mediating mechanism of sustainable performance.

Acquisition and improvement of mediating mechanisms: an example from the sport of cycling

In many ways, skill development in medical practice is like strength and conditioning training in sport; it occurs through the acquisition and improvement of mediating mechanisms. Take the sport of cycling, for example. Cycling can be performed on the road, in an arena, on off-road mountain bike trails or through a BMX obstacle course.

It can be done as an individual or as part of a peloton. All types of cycling draw on muscle groups to propel forward and navigate obstacles. The choice of muscle groups and the way each are deliberately deployed creates significant differences in the results produced, in terms of key performance indicators for the sport such as speed, endurance and safety. If the surface is damp, adjustments are made to maximise traction on the road. Cognitive mechanisms control the performance (e.g. deciding which muscle groups to deploy in order to achieve the desired result in the performance conditions), and physiological mechanisms execute the performance (e.g. posture and the movements of muscle groups). Results are produced with gradual and persistent training of aspects of performance, under particular conditions of the road and environment. To maintain a certain level of performance, ongoing practice is required.

In addition to the ability-related mediators of performance (e.g. strength and fitness), trait-related and other mediators of performance are necessary (e.g. drive and determination). If the cyclist has the capability to cycle, but has no desire or motivation to do so and chooses to sleep in, performance does not occur.

Common mediating mechanisms associated with increased levels of performance

Studies of expert-novice differences have revealed a range of mediating mechanisms associated with increased levels of performance, particularly knowledge and memory structures. Feltovich, Prietula and Ericsson (2006) state that "experts restructure, reorganise and refine their representation of knowledge and procedures for efficient application to their work-a-day environments" (p. 57). Additionally, experts tend to show long-term retention for domain-related material, can retrieve knowledge quickly from long-term memory, and have complex patterns in memory for recognising and responding to stimuli (Feltovich, Prietula & Ericsson, 2006). Experts' knowledge and memory structures provide them with a ready reference point for anticipating and responding to stimuli.

Deliberate practice

"'The aspiring expert performer needs to be able to find ways to go beyond their current state of maximal performance and find a way through training to improve the mediating mechanisms.''
(Ericsson, 2009, p. 415)

Deliberate practice is a specialised form of practice that allows the incremental developmental process to occur. It is based on the premise that the human body and brain respond to challenges by developing new abilities, and it works by harnessing the adaptability of brain and body to create the ability to do things previously not possible, one step at a time (Ericsson, 2016). Ericsson's principles of deliberate practice include:

- breaking learning down into a series of defined skills, levels or steps
- designing exercises to teach each of those skills, levels or steps in the correct order
- monitoring progress and giving immediate feedback on performance
- allowing for repetition and adjustment of performance with feedback.

One of the main purposes of deliberate practice is to develop a set of effective mental representations that can guide the mentee's performance of a skill. Mental representations are patterns of information held in long-term memory (e.g. images, facts, rules, relationships) that serve as mental shortcuts and make it possible to overcome the limitations of short-term memory. Mental representations are built by trying to perform a skill, adjusting the performance to be closer to the desired result, and trying again, over and over. For the mentee, the key benefit of mental representations is how they help to deal with information, for example, understanding and interpreting it, retaining it in memory, organising it, analysing it, making decisions with it, and assimilating new information. Mental representations provide an understanding of what a skill should look and feel like at every moment, enabling the mentee to produce and control their body movements, and monitor and correct their performance of the skill. In building mental representations, the mentee absorbs information connected with that skill, which helps the mentee to develop other skills (Ericsson, 2015; Ericsson, 2016).

Tips for assisting the mentee to acquire and improve a skill, based on the principles of deliberate practice, include:

- demonstrating how to perform the skill
- teaching the steps of the skill or technique in the correct order
- identifying errors that the mentee is making in their performance of the skill and giving immediate feedback
- guiding the mentee in recognising good performance
- designing practice activities for correcting errors, overcoming limitations and reaching the next level of performance
- encouraging the mentee to attempt performance of a skill that is not easy for them, under appropriate supervision (Ericsson, 2016).

The expert-performance approach

The expert-performance approach is a systematic way of examining and fostering the development of expertise in relation to a specific skill or task. It is useful for understanding the cognitive and physiological mediating mechanisms responsible for performance, and for designing methods of maintaining and improving performance of the skill or task through the acquisition of cognitive and physiological mediating mechanisms (Ericsson, 2006; Ericsson, 2007; Ericsson, 2015).

> "The expert-performance approach with deliberate practice is in many respects
> the opposite of general education because it starts by focussing specifically
> on the particular desired end product of training and experience – namely the
> representative target performance of medical specialists, such as surgeons
> or radiologists who have patient outcomes that are superior to their peers...
> the expert-performance approach includes an attempt to assess participants'
> thought processes and involves evaluating how the improved performance is
> mediated through and integrated with other skills and knowledge related to
> the final or target superior professional performance."
> (Ericsson, 2015, p. 1476)

The expert-performance approach encompasses analysis of mechanisms that mediate superior performance of the skill or task in representative task conditions, design of training that enables reproduction of the superior performance, and repetition of performance with detection and correction of errors.

Appendix B
The developmental journey of a doctor

Acquisition and improvement of mediating mechanisms for roles and tasks of the doctor in practice

Returning to the CanMEDS Framework, the roles of a doctor are communicator, collaborator, leader, health advocate, scholar, professional, and the integrating role of medical expert (Frank, Snell & Sherbino, 2015). Associated with each of these roles are competencies linked to essential tasks of practice. Building on Figure A1, p.192, Figure B1 represents in a very broad sense the doctor's potential acquisition of mediating mechanisms associated with improvement in their performance of essential tasks within each of the CanMEDS roles. (The position of roles on the graph is arbitrary, for illustrative purposes only.)

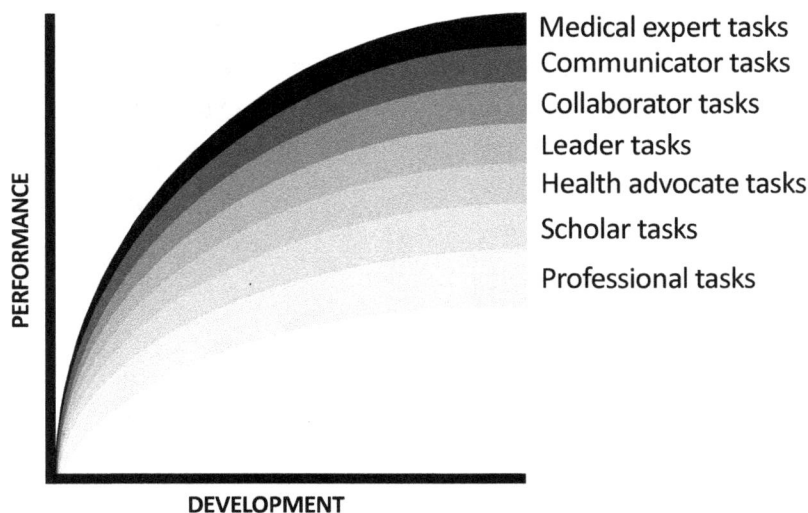

Figure B1. Developing performance of the doctor's roles
Adapted from Ericsson (2006)

A journey of transformation over time

The acquisition of mediating mechanisms associated with improving performance as a doctor is like a journey of transformation over time. Aspirational states of developments are milestones along the way. The portion of the journey from intern to consultant (approximately eight to ten years) starts with the doctor possessing smaller and simpler sets of mediating mechanisms, producing a repertoire of knowing, doing and being at intern level. Ideally, it culminates in the doctor possessing larger and more complex sets of mediating mechanisms, producing a repertoire of knowing, doing and being at consultant level. The journey of transformation does not end with the completion of clinical training; all doctors must continue to adapt within the complex adaptive system of healthcare.

Tracking development with developmental scales and frameworks

Developmental scales and frameworks provide signposts for the mentee on their developmental journey, and for those who support them. With varying degrees of specificity, the scales and frameworks turn something abstract, the notion of a developmental journey, into something more solid, for example, a set of knowledge, skills and behaviours for the mentee to acquire, and milestones to reach. Table B1 features prominent developmental scales and frameworks.

Table B1. Developmental scales and frameworks

DEVELOPMENTAL SCALE	ORIGINATOR	QUALITATIVE MEASURES AND DESCRIPTION
Millers Pyramid	Miller (Miller, 1990)	A framework for the assessment of clinical skills, competence and performance at the levels of knows, knows how, shows how and does
The conscious competence learning model	Broadwell, (Broadwell, 1969)	Competence development, over stages of unconscious incompetence, conscious incompetence, conscious competence and unconscious competence
RIME	Pangaro (Pangaro, 1999)	A system of assessing the doctor's level of information processing at the levels of Reporter, Interpreter, Manager and Educator
Skill acquisition	Dreyfus (Leach, 2002; Leach, 2004)	Moving from rule-based behaviours to context-based behaviours through the stages of novice, advanced beginner, competent, proficient, expert and master
Phases of practitioner development	Skovholt and Trotter-Mathison (2016)	Developing as a practitioner through the phases of lay helper, beginning student, advanced student, novice professional, experienced professional and senior professional.
Draft CanMEDS 2015 Milestones Guide	Royal College of Physicians and Surgeons of Canada (Frank, Snell, Sherbino, et al., 2014)	Milestones to meet at levels of requirements for residency, transition to discipline, foundations of discipline, core of discipline, transition to practice and advanced expertise
JDocs framework	Royal Australasian College of Surgeons (RACS, 2016)	Tasks, skills and behaviours that should be achieved by doctors at defined, early postgraduate year levels, and will assist in their development towards a career in surgery and other proceduralist careers

Appendix C
Guiding reflective enquiry

Sample reflective enquiry prompts

Table C1 includes prompts for the mentee's reflective enquiry across the three dimensions of development, knowing, doing and being, organised by when the reflective enquiry occurs. Schön's work (1983) (as cited by Ryan, 2010), describes four categories of reflective enquiry: reflection before action, knowing in action, reflection in action and reflection on action. *Reflection before action* happens while moving towards an encounter with a patient and involves anticipating the encounter, recalling relevant learning from experience that may be applicable to the encounter, and checking one's mood and energy in preparation for the anticipated encounter. *Knowing in action* happens in the moment of the encounter, thinking and reacting in a fast and unconscious way. *Reflection in action* involves critical thinking and making informed, rational decisions linked to reflection during the encounter. *Reflection on action* is looking back on the encounter afterwards, in order to find lessons for future practice.

While these prompts are framed as questions that the mentee can use for their own reflective enquiry, they can be translated into questions that the mentor uses with the mentee to guide and or teach reflective enquiry.

Table C1. Reflective enquiry prompts

REFLECTIVE ENQUIRY		
KNOWING	**DOING**	**BEING**
What do I learn easily?	*Reflection in action.*	What preconceptions, assumptions, biases and beliefs do I hold that are relevant to patient care?
What do I find most challenging to learn?	What patient cues are concerning?	
What learning strategies work best for me to make learning stick?	What immediate adjustments do I need to make in my practice?	What is my concept of 'who I am as a doctor'?
What are my attitudes towards lifelong learning?	Are there ethical issues? What are they?	Who do I want to become as a doctor?
How can I embed lifelong learning in my practice?	Are there value conflicts What are they?	Who do I not want to become as a doctor?
How is my knowledge structured?	What would this situation look like if I was managing it effectively?	What are my authentic values?
		How do I prioritise my values?
What feedback have I received about my knowledge base?	What am I assuming about this situation that may be incorrect?	How do I voice my values?
What will I do with what I know?	How are my past experiences influencing my responses now?	How do I resolve value conflicts?
Reflection before action.		How well are my personal values integrated with values of the profession?
Where are the gaps in my knowledge and skill base?	*Reflection on action.*	
	What theories, concepts and rules guided me in this situation?	How do I balance self-care with other-care?
How will I know when I am out of my depth?	How did I know to take action?	What did I learn about myself?
When will I need to call for help?	What cues did I respond to?	How willing am I to receive constructive feedback with an open mind?
Where will I find help?	What gave me a sense of confusion?	
	What were my reactions?	How important is it to me to have insight?
	What were the implications of my reactions for the patient?	
	What did I do and what resulted?	
	What moral and ethical criteria did I apply?	
	Has my perspective of patient care changed?	
	What was significant about the situation?	
	Did I think about how the patient feels?	

Fostering metacognition

One of the core aims of medical education is to help the doctor acquire expertise. In decades past this was thought to be a relatively straightforward process of possessing a great deal of subject knowledge and seeing many different patient presentations. The huge increase in medical knowledge, which more than doubles every five years, has outstripped the capacity of the human brain to absorb it (Eichbaum, 2014; Robinson, 1993). This vast increase in knowledge is made more overwhelming by the fact that approximately 90% of this information becomes outdated or redundant ten years after publication (Robinson, 1993). To become an expert in today's medical workplace the doctor needs to develop the ability to assimilate new knowledge, experience and skills throughout their working life and to be continually adapting, changing and growing the way they think and practice. This capacity is driven by a combination of the clinician's metacognitive capabilities and deliberate practice (Ericsson, 2004; Quirk, 2006).

Metacognition is a type of reflective practice that can be thought of as "thinking about your thinking". Drilling down further as to what that actually means, we need to look at the academic literature where it is described as any knowledge or cognitive process that monitors or controls your thinking. There are two broad divisions of metacognition: knowing about cognition and regulation of cognition (Flavell, 1987). The knowledge of cognition component includes knowing about one's intellectual capabilities, knowing how to implement learning strategies and knowing when and why to use these learning techniques. The regulation of cognition consists of planning, selective focusing, monitoring one's learning strategies and debugging strategies used to correct performance errors and analyse performance.

Metacognition in medical practice is like a steering wheel for thinking and learning. Doctors need to know what the steering wheel is capable of and how to use it to drive their thinking and learning successfully. Metacognition is essential for sound clinical reasoning because the clinical reasoning process is steered by the doctor's metacognitive skills engaging with their cognitive capabilities and the knowledge that they acquire. These metacognitive skills monitor the information being received, and help the doctor recruit specific cognitive processes as well as memories, to determine their next course of action (Colbert et al., 2015). This course of action can include identifying the next piece of information to look for, or determining if they have sufficient information to be confident in making a decision.

At a practical level, it is helpful to know how to grow these metacognitive skills both for ourselves as well as those we may mentor. There are two complimentary approaches that work well to grow a culture where metacognitive skills can develop and thrive. Explicitly teaching metacognitive skills is one approach that brings into sharp focus the need of the mentee to think about their own thinking (Pintrich, 2002). For example, to highlight the importance of planning, which is part of regulating metacognition, a mentor may ask the mentee to reflect on what they already know about a topic or how are they going to actively scrutinise their own learning. Knowing about the importance of metacognitive 'monitoring' a mentor may ask the mentee if they can distinguish important information from detail, and if not how will they will figure out the difference. In the 'evaluating' component of metacognition the mentor may ask the mentee what they learned today that conflicted with their prior understanding or what was the most confusing aspect of what they learned today (Tanner, 2012).

A second, effective way to develop metacognition within the clinical workplace is to intentionally grow a learning environment that is supportive of metacognition. One way of doing this is for the mentor to actively role model their own metacognitive processes. In doing so, the mentee starts to anticipate what they will see, experience and reflect upon. The POSE mnemonic is a helpful way for the mentor to model their metacognition through a sequence of previewing, outlining, sharing and evaluating a case (Quirk, 2006, p. 107), *see* Appendix I, p.226.

Junior doctors, although high academic achievers, are not generally trained as critical thinkers, which is a vital aspect of clinical practice (Eichbaum, 2014). Developing metacognitive skills is essential in clinical decision making as well as navigating the sheer volume of medical knowledge being produced today.

Appendix D
The intentional mentor's job description

The work of the intentional mentor

Do relational work
Be trustworthy
CARE, be committed, accessible, responsive and engaged
Accept responsibilities, fulfil commitments, and adjust the partnership as the mentee develops or as circumstances change

Do developmental work
Contribute to the mentee's development as a doctor in practice

- Assist the mentee to acquire relevant knowledge and skills, performance, and awareness and practise of values
- Make every day work practices visible
- Make influences on work performance visible
- Encourage job knowledge and tacit knowledge gains
- Provide practice opportunities for situated learning
- Guide reflective enquiry
- Assist at points of transition
- Advocate

Assist the mentee with goal setting and achievement aligned with their aspirational state of development

- Help the mentee to figure out their aspirational state of development
- Assist the mentee to translate their aspirational state of development to goals
- Recognise and respond to the developmental needs of the mentee (for support, challenge and facilitation) in service of their goals
- Share work with the mentee: understand mentoring responsibilities and goals, have goal-directed interactions, and fulfil commitments

Give structure to mentoring

- Oversee the formation of the partnership, the collaboration and the parting of ways at the conclusion of mentoring (structuring the mentoring partnership)
- Oversee the mentee's goal setting and achievement (structuring the mentoring process for development)

Knowledge required

Relational work

- The importance of commitment, accessibility, responsiveness and engagement in building relationship
- Staging of the partnership over the course of mentoring

Developmental work

- The work of a doctor in practice
- Dimensions of doctor development – knowing, doing and being
- Support, challenge and facilitation as types of influence exerted by the mentor to foster development
- The concept of aspirational state of development as an ideal repertoire of knowing (a dynamic knowledge and skills base), doing (a set of performance behaviours) and being (awareness and practise of values)
- The connection between an aspirational state of development and learning, performance and values-related goals
- Recognising and responding to mentees' needs for support, challenge and facilitation in service of their goals
- How to have goal-directed interactions in mentoring including conversation-based and action-based activities
- Mentoring evaluation using process and outcome evaluation[*]
- Reflective practice of mentoring[*]

*Also part of the relational work of mentoring

Skills required

- Send and receive messages for particular purposes in mentoring, using listening, questioning and informing (use a relating and developing tool)
- Engage with the mentee for the duration of mentoring and link the mentee to the broader community of practice (use a connecting tool)
- Enhance the mentee's success in setting and achieving goals, and realising their aspirational state of development (use a progress tool)
- Identify competency areas and standards of performance relevant to the mentee's practice (use a focusing tool)
- Help the mentee overcome obstacles and accelerate their progress towards goal achievement (use an accelerating tool)
- Engage with the mentee in relation to impacts of work and how to turn stress into adaptation (use a fortifying tool)
- Orient the mentee towards useful resources, actions and decisions in relation to career (use a navigating tool)
- Protect confidential information shared during mentoring (use a safety tool)
- Identity the mentee's response to mentoring and progress attributable to mentoring (use a discovery tool)
- Learn mentoring from experience (use a self-monitoring tool)

Attributes

- Willingness to do relational and developmental work, and having goodwill
- Positive role modeling
- Genuineness
- Sound performance and participation in continuing professional development
- Possessing sound mentoring knowledge and skills

Performance indicators

Relational work – Mentor demonstrates CARE, commitment, accessibility, responsiveness and engagement

Developmental work – Mentor assists the mentee to set and achieve learning, performance and values-related goals aligned with the mentee's aspirational state of development

A metaphor for the mentor role

For those who enjoy metaphors, parallels exist between the mentor and the belayer in rock climbing. The belayer is the one who stand at the foot of the rock and controls the ropes for the climber. An understanding of the belayer role to a rock climber, can be translated into lessons about the mentor role, in preparation for taking on a mentor role. Table D1 draws the parallels.

Table D1. The belayer role in rock climber training as a metaphor for the mentor role in mentoring

THE BELAYER ROLE IN ROCK CLIMBING	TRANSLATING THE METAPHOR: THE MENTOR ROLE IN MENTORING
What is rock climber training?	**What is intentional mentoring?**
Rock climber training is a purpose-driven:	Mentoring is a purpose-driven:
partnership – two people in partnership (rock climber and belayer) who have a shared commitment to the rock climber's development and safety	partnership – a voluntary collaboration between two doctors with a difference in experience (mentor and mentee) who have a shared commitment to the junior doctor's (the mentee's) development
process – working together so that the climber can safely strive for gains in what they know and do and how they embody values and qualities of a rock climber, and move towards their aspirational state of development	process – working together so that the mentee can safely strive for gains in what they know and do and how they embody values and qualities of a doctor, and move towards their aspirational state of development
What is the belayer's role?	**What is the mentor's role?**
Half of the partnership and process (the helper's half)	Half of the partnership and process (the helper's half)
Relational work – commitment, responsibility, accessibility, engagement (CARE); staging (especially building trust initially)	Relational work – CARE; staging – empathic attachment, active involvement and felt separation
Developmental work – helping the climber to visualise a way of functioning, discussing goals for the climber's progress towards the desired functioning, contributing to the climber's goal achievement	Developmental work – assisting the mentee to identify their aspirational state of development, translating it to goals, then having goal-directed interactions
Contributing various forms of challenge, support and facilitation as part of the relational work and developmental work e.g. giving perspective and feedback on balance and breadth of developmental pursuits, and integration; helping the climber to set their sights, find their feet, get a feel for the terrain, find their way, and find their sense of self as a climber	Contributing various forms of challenge, support and facilitation as part of the relational work and developmental work
	Helping the mentee to set their sights, find their feet, get a feel for the terrain, find their way, and find their sense of self as a doctor

What should the belayer know, do and be, in their role?	What should the mentor know, do and be, in their role?
Know – what the climber should know, do and be as a rock climber to function effectively in their environment; what the climber needs in order to develop; techniques for building relationship and helping the rock climber to develop	Know – what the mentee should know, do and be as a doctor to function effectively in their context; what the mentee needs in order to develop; techniques for building relationship and helping the mentee to develop
Do – rock climbing practice to understand what is involved in the sport and how to be an effective belayer; staging partnership and building trust, applying influence (challenge, support and facilitation), and keeping sight of the focal points of the work (relational work and developmental work)	Do – medical practice and own development as a doctor; mentoring practice in mentor role: staging mentoring (empathic attachment, active involvement and felt separation), applying influence (challenge, support and facilitation), and keeping sight of the focal points of the work (relational work and developmental work)
Be – functional, careful, detail-oriented and patient in order to maximise safety for the climber	Be – functional, genuine, believing that others deserve CARE
Tools to develop and use in the belayer role	**Tools to develop and use in the mentor role**
Purposeful communication	Purposeful communication
Partnership	Partnership
Goal-directed interaction	Goal-directed interaction
Brief intervention	Curriculum and performance standards
Resilience work	Brief intervention
Evaluation	Resilience work
	Career guidance
	Confidentiality
	Reflective practice of mentoring
	Evaluation
Special issues to give attention to	**Special issues to give attention to**
Transition to a new level of challenge	Transition to a new job or level of seniority
Aspirations for pursuing the sport	Aspirations for pursuing a career path
Resilience including building strength and flexibility	Resilience including stress and energy management and self-preservation
	Addressing bullying (if applicable)

Appendix E
The making of the Model of Intentional Mentoring, I-Mentor with the Cycle of Caring and the intentional mentor's toolkit

This section explains how the Model of Intentional Mentoring, I-Mentor with the Cycle of Caring, and the intentional mentor's toolkit were generated, as shown in Figure E1.

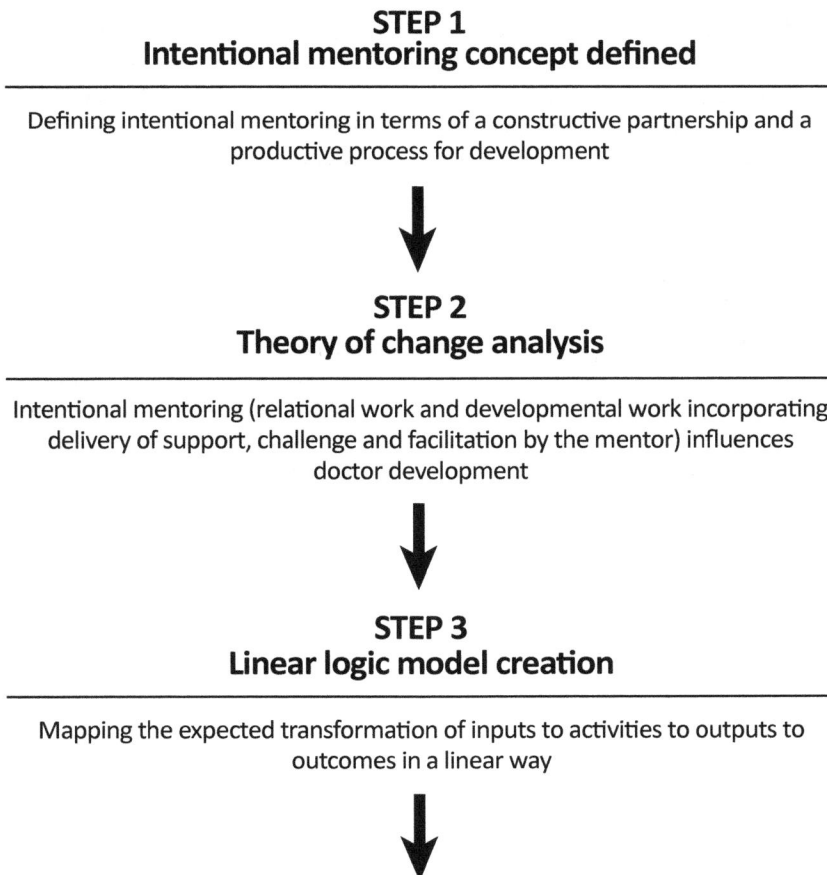

STEP 1
Intentional mentoring concept defined

Defining intentional mentoring in terms of a constructive partnership and a productive process for development

↓

STEP 2
Theory of change analysis

Intentional mentoring (relational work and developmental work incorporating delivery of support, challenge and facilitation by the mentor) influences doctor development

↓

STEP 3
Linear logic model creation

Mapping the expected transformation of inputs to activities to outputs to outcomes in a linear way

↓

$$\downarrow$$

STEP 4
Cyclic logic model creation

Mapping the expected transformation of inputs to activities to outputs to outcomes in a cyclic way that incorporates feedback
The model is named the Model of Intentional Mentoring

$$\downarrow$$

STEP 5
Revealing the mentor's role in intentional mentoring

An approach to the mentor's role is created through combining the Model of Intentional Mentoring with the Cycle of Caring (Skovholt, 2005)
The model for the mentor's role is named I-Mentor with the Cycle of Caring

$$\downarrow$$

STEP 6
Identifying ten tools of the intentional mentor

The tools enable the mentor to build relationship and foster development using support, challenge and facilitation
Collectively the tools are known as the intentional mentor's toolkit

Figure E1. The making of the Model of Intentional Mentoring, I-Mentor with the Cycle of Caring and the intentional mentor's toolkit

Appendix F
Communication basics refresher

Verbals and non-verbals

Communication between two people is often deconstructed to activities of a sender (a speaker) and a receiver (a listener) sending and receiving messages in an orderly fashion. This type of deconstruction belies the complexity of what is simultaneously going on in the exchange, verbally and non-verbally. In an exchange, both speaker and listener are simultaneously sending and receiving non-verbal messages, while the speaker sends and the listener receives a verbal message. Mehrabian (1981) studied the communication of feelings and attitudes and quantified how much liking is conveyed in words and non-verbal cues. His findings were: 7% for words spoken; 38% for the way the words are said; and 55% for facial expressions. These results have implications for the mentor role relating to the power of non-verbal cues in conveying feelings and attitudes. Being aware of what you are communicating non-verbally, and taking care to ensure congruence of your words and non-verbal cues, improves communication.

Essential communication ingredients

Active listening

Active listening is comprised of three main parts (Kotzman, 1989):
1. Attending – paying attention to all verbal and non-verbal cues in the exchange of communication.
2. Following – following where the mentee is taking you, without trying to direct the flow of the communication.
3. Reflecting – confirming your understanding of what you have heard the mentee say through paraphrasing and summarising. Your reflecting may focus on content (the key meaning of what was said) or feeling (the emotion conveyed in the message).

Questioning

To invite an *amount* of information and detail, categories of questions are:

- open questions to invite detailed, lengthy answers
- closed questions to invite short, direct answers.

To elicit a *type* of information and detail, categories of questions are:

- objective questions to elicit data, facts and sensory information
- reflective questions to elicit to personal reactions and associations
- interpretive questions to elicit meaning, significance and implications
- decisional questions to elicit resolutions for the future (Spencer, 1989).

Informing

According to Knowles' (1984) adult learning principles, information that is delivered should:

- give the mentee choice in what is discussed, and the responsibility for their own learning
- build on the mentee's existing knowledge and skills
- connect to the mentee's roles and tasks
- be useful now
- connect with and stimulate the mentee's interests (*see* Appendix H, pp.219–23).

Appendix G
Persuasive communication

The Rhetorical Triangle

The Rhetorical Triangle (Ramage, Bean & Johnson, 2012) is an approach to persuasive communication that applies within mentoring conversations. To take this approach, first figure out what the purpose of your message is, considering questions such as: What statement do I wish to make? What effect would I like to have? What movement or momentum am I hoping to create? Ideally, the purpose of your message fits with the bigger picture of the mentee's goals. After figuring out the purpose of your message, use three kinds of persuasive appeals to deliver the message for maximum impact: *logos*, ensuring the content of the conversation is sequenced in a logical way, *ethos*, choosing how to present yourself as a voice of authority and a credible source of information, and *pathos*, showing an understanding of the mentee's beliefs and values, and appealing to their emotions and imagination. Persuasive communication using the three appeals is illustrated in Figure G1.

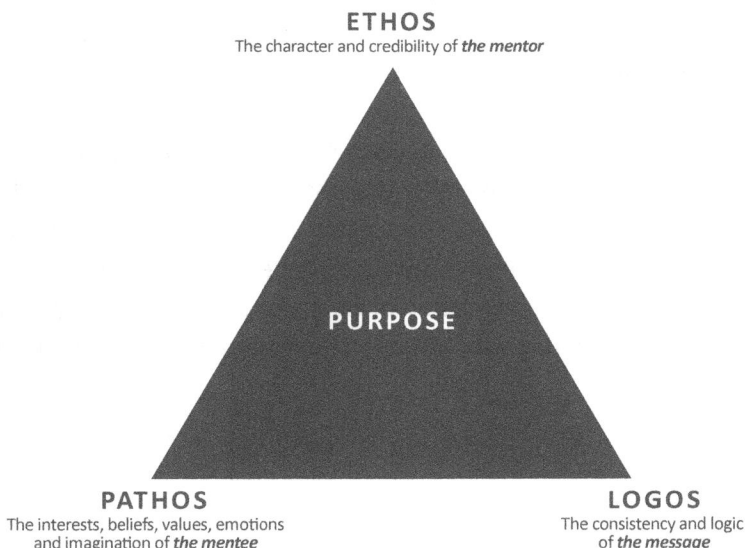

ETHOS
The character and credibility of *the mentor*

PURPOSE

PATHOS
The interests, beliefs, values, emotions
and imagination of *the mentee*

LOGOS
The consistency and logic
of *the message*

Figure G1. The three appeals of The Rhetorical Triangle in mentoring
Adapted from: Ramage, Bean & Johnson (2012)

In a medicine, *pathos* relates to baseline knowledge of an audience. If a haematologist gives a talk to fellow haematologists about lymphoma, they share extensive baseline knowledge about the subject. A lot of information is assumed knowledge. Because the baseline knowledge is high, the content is more detailed. However, if the same haematologist is asked to talk about lymphoma to a group of patients, the baseline knowledge of the group is likely to be lower. The haematologist's content has to change or it will be irrelevant to the patients. Doctors frequently err on the side of high assumed baseline knowledge when they should err on the side of low assumed baseline knowledge. This is because most people are more comfortable talking about and teaching something that they are more familiar with. It is also easy to forget what not knowing is like.

In a mentoring context, understanding the mentee through listening and questioning allows you to identify the mentee's baseline knowledge, structure content logically and pitch it at an appropriate level, and present yourself as a credible, trustworthy source of information. By attending to *logos*, *pathos* and *ethos,* communication with your mentee is more likely to reach them and inspire them to action. Tips for applying *logos*, *pathos* and *ethos* follow, incorporating ideas from Ramage, Bean and Johnson (2012).

Logos, appealing with logic

- Give a reference point. What does the topic have to do with the mentee's goals? How does the subject build on something discussed previously? Is there a previous reference point? Contextualise, e.g. "This follows on from..."
- Explain your reasoning. Convey to the mentee why you think what you think and how you have arrived at certain ideas, identifying and revealing assumptions if there is a possibility that assumptions are not shared.
- Sequence information logically. Pre-existing formats or frameworks may be useful as a guide in certain circumstances. An example of a pre-existing formula for logos that enables transmission of clear, concise and logically sequenced information, is ISBAR (Identify, Situation, Background, Assessment and Recommendation).

Ethos, revealing your character and establishing credibility

- Reveal persona. Persona refers to aspects of your personality that you present to others. Decide which aspect or aspects of yourself you are most comfortable revealing to the mentee, and which ones help you to function most effectively in your mentor role.
- Find and use your voice as a mentor. Voice refers to your distinctive style of expression. Your use of voice may differ depending on the activity and context you are in. For example, the voice of authority that you use at home as a parent is likely to differ from the voice of authority that you use at work as a doctor or a mentor.
- Build trust through shared values. Conveying values that you share with the mentee can be a basis for building trust and finding common ground.
- Be knowledgeable. Draw from examples, experiences, statistics and reliable data sources to make your case.
- Be fair. Show that you empathise with other points of views and demonstrate a courteous attitude to opposing views.

Pathos, engaging the mentee's feelings and imagination

- Reveal your understanding of the world of the mentee. Acknowledge parts of the mentee's life that they are passionate and emotive about, or interested in. Connect your message with those parts of the mentee's life.
- Ensure relevance of your message to the mentee. When responding to a question from the mentee, answer the question to the best of your ability and confirm with them that you have answered their question fully.
- Use concrete language, examples, illustrations, narratives, metaphors and analogies that appeal to the mentee's emotions and imagination.

Appendix H
Principles and practices of teaching and giving feedback

Teaching knowledge and skills

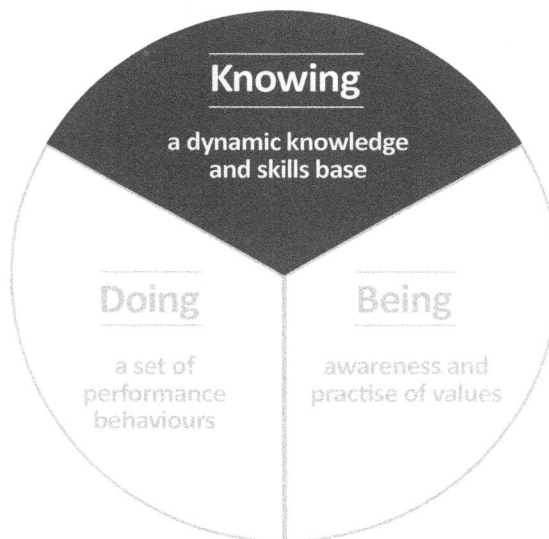

Knowing
a dynamic knowledge and skills base

Doing
a set of performance behaviours

Being
awareness and practise of values

Knowles' (1984) five assumptions about the characteristics of adult learners are the basis of andragogy, the art and science of helping adults learn, and can guide episodes of teaching knowledge and skills. Table H4 converts the assumptions to implications for teaching, and teaching practice examples. Our view of the importance of integrating knowing, doing and being in the medical profession aligns with Knowles' work.

Table H1. Principles and practices of teaching adults

ASSUMPTIONS ABOUT THE CHARACTERISTICS OF ADULT LEARNERS	IMPLICATIONS FOR TEACHING	EXAMPLES OF TEACHING PRACTICES
Self-concept: As a person matures his/her self-concept moves from one of being a dependent personality toward one of being a self-directed human being	Teaching gives freedom, choice and responsibility	Giving the mentee responsibility for their learning
		Creating learning experiences that allow autonomy
		Offering guidance, availability to respond to questions, and assistance with overcoming obstacles, but letting the mentee learn on their own terms
		Allowing the mentee to have an active contribution to the educational process
		Giving the mentee choice in teaching and learning methods
		Involving the mentee in planning learning experiences
		Encouraging the mentee to identify and utilise learning resources
		Providing more support at the start and less support as the mentee becomes self-directed
		Allowing the mentee the freedom to develop their own style of learning
		Encouraging the mentee to self-assess
		Creating a learning environment that encourages freedom of expression
Experience: As a person matures he/she accumulates a growing reservoir of experience that becomes an increasing resource for learning	Teaching builds on existing knowledge and skills	Recognising diversity in backgrounds, experiences and skills sets, that affect learning
		Establishing the mentee's existing knowledge and skills through dialogue and observation
		Finding reference points in the mentee's experience that will connect with the teaching content
		Identifying the mentee's knowledge gaps
		Demonstrating respect for the mentee's experiences, accomplishments, and starting point for new knowledge and skills
		Offering activities that involve experience, repetition and constructive feedback
		Allowing experience, including mistakes, to be a basis for teaching

Readiness to learn:	Teaching connects to roles and tasks	Conveying the applications of the new information and ideas
As a person matures his/her readiness to learn becomes oriented increasingly to the developmental tasks of his social roles		Assisting the mentee to fine tune their skills for roles
		Providing learning opportunities that are task-oriented
		Providing opportunities and support for practice
		Describing how the lessons can be applied in solving problems faced in practice
		Including real world examples, scenarios and role plays
Orientation to learning:	Teaching is useful now	Assisting the mentee to appreciate the immediate relevance of the new information
As a person matures his/her time perspective changes from one of postponed application of knowledge to immediacy of application, and accordingly his/her orientation toward learning shifts from one of subject-centeredness to one of problem- centredness		Conveying the immediate relevance of the lesson to a healthcare problem that the mentee is responsible for solving in their job
		Offering problem-centred and problem-based learning
		Designing problem solving activities as part of the learning process
		Explaining why the mentee needs to learn the lesson
		Using stories to illustrate the relevance of the lesson
		Explaining how the new information will help the mentee to solve problems
		Giving examples of how the new knowledge and skills can be applied now
Motivation to learn:	Teaching connects with and stimulates interests	Identifying the mentee's interests and emotions, and linking these to the mentee's learning
As a person matures the motivation to learn is internal		Seeking to motivate the mentee
		Helping the mentee to tap into their intrinsic motivation
		Helping the mentee to find meaning in what they are learning
		Giving the mentee a relevant reason for completing the learning activities
		Leveraging the mentee's desire to do the best for the patient
		Using interesting clinical cases to stimulate the mentee's desire to learn

Source: Knowles (1984)

Giving feedback on performance (feedback on doing)

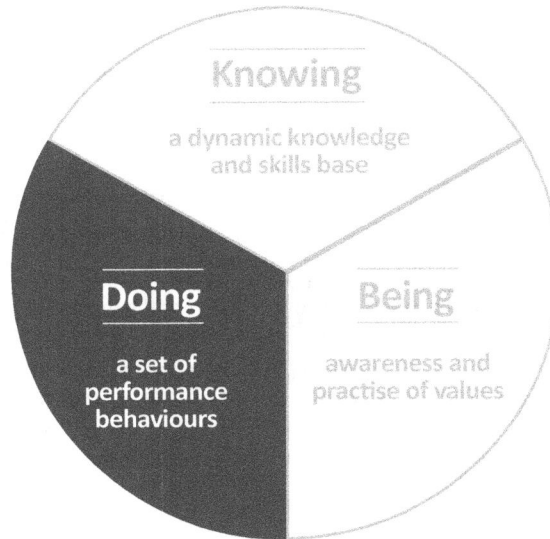

The object of giving feedback on performance is to close the gap between actual and desired performance. Giving feedback is teaching in response to performance, to assist the mentee to achieve their performance goals. As such, Knowles' (1984) five assumptions of characteristics of adult learners can be used to organise an approach to giving feedback on performance. Table H2 displays examples of feedback practices based on the work of Ende (1983).

Table H2. Principles and practices of giving feedback on performance

ASSUMPTIONS ABOUT THE CHARACTERISTICS OF ADULT LEARNERS	IMPLICATIONS FOR GIVING FEEDBACK ON PERFORMANCE	EXAMPLES OF FEEDBACK PRACTICES
Self-concept: As a person matures his/her self-concept moves from one of being a dependent personality toward one of being a self-directed human being	Feedback gives freedom, choice and responsibility	Giving the mentee choice in relation to aspects of the delivery of the feedback (e.g. the time and place, to uphold confidentiality and avoid humiliating the mentee) Delivering feedback as part of dialogue with the mentee

Experience: As a person matures he/she accumulates a growing reservoir of experience that becomes an increasing resource for learning	Feedback builds on existing knowledge and skills	Showing respect for the mentee's experiences and efforts
		Basing feedback on a credible source of information, preferably direct observation
		Checking the mentee's insight into the quality of their performance by asking the mentee for their impressions
		Responding to the mentee's impressions respectfully
		For areas requiring improvement, asking the mentee how they feel they can improve, to allow them to arrive at a breakthrough, before giving your feedback
		Referring to standards or criteria applied in assessing the performance
		Translating observations into a description of specific behaviours relative to a standard
		Giving feedback in digestible amounts
		Asking the mentee to summarise their understanding of the feedback provided
Readiness to learn: As a person matures his/her readiness to learn becomes oriented increasingly to the developmental tasks of his social roles	Feedback connects to roles and tasks	Giving feedback that relates to aspects of performance that are most important to roles and essential tasks
		Clearly conveying the aspects performed well, and aspects that were overlooked or that need improvement
		Describing the behaviours to continue and discontinue
Orientation to learning: As a person matures his/her time perspective changes from one of postponed application of knowledge to immediacy of application, and accordingly his/her orientation toward learning shifts from one of subject-centeredness to one of problem-centredness	Feedback is useful now	Taking advantage of teachable moments, at the time of the performance or shortly after
		Including a plan for applying the new knowledge or behaviour at work as soon as possible
Motivation to learn: As a person matures the motivation to learn is internal	Feedback connects with and stimulates interests	Recognising that the mentee may be apprehensive about receiving feedback
		Increasing the mentee's receptivity to feedback by presenting feedback as a normal component of teaching; teaching occurs, learning is demonstrated and assessed, and assessment findings are shared as feedback
		Providing feedback on aspects of performance that interest the mentee
		Delivering feedback calmly and sensitively
		Avoiding humiliating the mentee

Source: Knowles (1984)

Giving values-focused feedback (feedback on being)

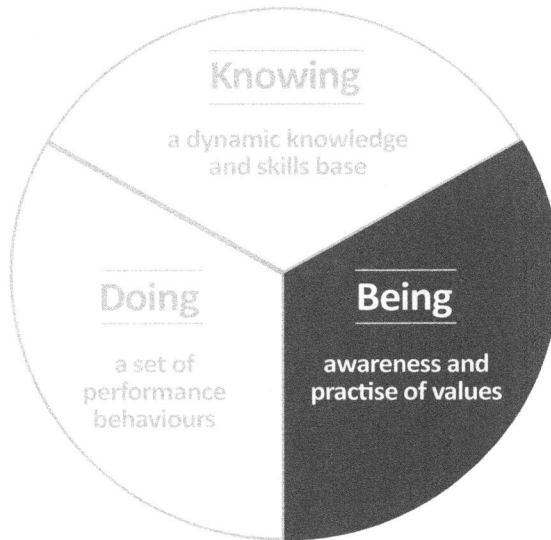

The object of values-focused feedback is to encourage the mentee's awareness and practise of personal and professional values. Table H3 displays steps and examples of feedback practices.

Table H3. Giving values-focused feedback

STEP	EXAMPLES OF FEEDBACK PRACTICES
Establish a values reference point	Identifying the mentee's core personal and professional values
Raise awareness of value conflicts and values-inconsistent actions	Identifying values in actions taken by the mentee Comparing values held and values enacted Identifying how values were prioritised or sacrificed Identifying incongruence in personal and professional values Identifying imbalance in science and humanistic values Encouraging perception of others' values (e.g. patients' and colleagues' values) and the priority they give to values
Reconcile values and prepare for future value conflicts	Noticing how competing ideals were resolved Identifying unresolved value conflicts Exploring how competing ideals might be resolved Exploring ways to further integrate personal and professional values Exploring ways to balance science and humanistic values Anticipating and discussing opportunities for enacting values in the future

Appendix I
Brief intervention frameworks

Brief intervention can help the mentee to make progress more quickly than would otherwise be possible in the time available, or to overcome a particular obstacle that is hindering their progress in goal achievement. Table I1 summarises a range of brief intervention frameworks loosely categorised by the dimensions of development, knowing, doing and being. For further explanations, refer to the source publications.

Table I1. Brief intervention frameworks

DIMENSION OF MENTEE'S DEVELOPMENT	FACILITATING THE MENTEE'S...	THEORY/ FRAMEWORK	DESCRIPTION
Knowing	Learning of knowledge	Peyton's Set, Dialogue and Closure (Lake & Ryan, 2004)	Planning and delivering teaching based on a triad of concepts: Set – forming clear, relevant and achievable learning outcomes for the time available Dialogue – engaging the learner with relevant content Closure – summarising take-home messages and linking learning to self-directed learning or future teaching
Knowing	Learning of a skill	Peyton's model (Lake & Hamdorf, 2004)	A sequence of demonstration and deconstruction of the skill (by the trainer) followed by comprehension and performance of the skill (by the learner)
Knowing	Learning of knowledge and clinical reasoning	One-Minute Preceptor (Neher, Gordon, Meyer & Stevens, 1992; Neher & Stevens, 2003)	Questioning and informing the mentee about a clinical care aspect of a case using five micro-skills: asking for a commitment to a diagnosis or a plan exploring supporting evidence teaching general rules verbally reinforcing effective actions correcting mistakes.

Knowing	Metacognition *see also* Appendix C, pp.203–4	Quirk (2006, p. 107)	POSE is a mnemonic to assist the mentor to model metacognition: P – Preview (identifying and naming any relevant information in readiness for meeting the patient, to help the mentee frame the next clinical case) O – Outline (outlining what you are about to experience, think or do, to give the mentee the chance to reflect on any thoughts or feelings that might influence their decisions or behaviours, such as the age or underlying co-morbidities of the patient) S – Share (sharing thoughts, feelings or concerns that might influence your decisions or behaviours, to give the mentee a greater awareness of what you regard as the important components of the patient case) E – Evaluate (evaluating the experience after it has taken place including a review of your behaviours, thoughts and feelings during and after the patient encounter, as well as those of the mentee)
Knowing and doing	Reflective practice	Gibbs' Reflective Cycle (Gibbs, 1988)	Guiding the mentee in reflecting on an experience of practice through six stages: description, feelings, evaluation, analysis, conclusion and action plan
Knowing and doing	Learning from experience	Debriefing with good judgment (Rudolph, Simon, Rivard, Dufresne & Raemer, 2007)	Giving constructive feedback, through surfacing assumptions and the open sharing of opinions or personal points of view. Assuming that the mentee is doing their best and that their responses deserve respect Helping the mentee to transform their mistakes into learning and merge experience with new knowledge
Knowing and Doing	Development of expertise	Cognitive apprenticeship (Collins, 2005)	A series of interactions, incorporating modelling, coaching, scaffolding, articulation, reflection and exploration
Doing	Receptivity to feedback and insight	The reflective feedback conversation (Cantillon & Sargeant, 2008)	Asking the mentee to share any concerns about their performance and to reflect on what might improve their performance, providing views on the performance, and correcting and checking for understanding
Doing	Identification of individual and environmental obstacles to practice	Gilbert's framework (Gilbert, 1978, Chapter 3)	Reviewing individual and environmental levels of influence in relation to performance, to identify problems to do with information, instrumentation or motivation

Doing	Action	Miracle question and exception finding, from Solution-focused therapy (De Jong & Berg, 2008)	Miracle question: asking the mentee to imagine in detail what they would be doing and how their work life would be more positive if problems/barriers to practice disappeared Exception finding: asking the mentee to identify past successes as possible exemplars of useful future action
Being	Awareness and practise of values	Giving Voice to Values (Ethics Unwrapped, 2016)	Enhancing the mentee's ability to voice and enact values, through helping them with: awareness of widely held 'universal values' of honesty, respect, fairness and compassion recognising the choice to act or not act on values realising that value conflicts are normal and predictable knowing what they are trying to accomplish and the impact they wish to have knowing what they believe in and stand for, and having a 'self-story' that gives encouragement and confidence practising phrases in advance for expressing values effectively preparing to encounter and respond to the most common values challenges at work.
Being	Mindfulness and values-focused action	STOP (Harris, 2007)	STOP is a mnemonic related to managing thoughts and feelings effectively, and taking helpful action: S – Slow down including slowing your breathing T – Take note of thoughts and feelings and what you are doing O – Open up to having thoughts and feelings just as they are P – Pursue values and let your values guide whatever you choose to do next

Appendix J
Frameworks for resilience and quality of life

A selection of evidence-based approaches to fostering resilience and quality of life is summarises in Table J1. While these approaches are commonly used as frameworks for counselling and coaching, they may also be sources of ideas for resilience work in mentoring for those readers wishing to acquire advanced skills.

Table J1. Frameworks for resilience and quality of life

EVIDENCE-BASED APPROACH	A PROBLEM, THROUGH THE LENS OF THE FRAMEWORK	A SOLUTION, THROUGH THE LENS OF THE FRAMEWORK
Acceptance and Commitment Therapy (Hayes & Smith, 2005)	Struggling with uncomfortable thought and feelings and not pursuing valued actions diminishes quality of life	Managing thoughts and feelings effectively and pursuing valued actions improves quality of life
Solution-focused therapy (De Jong & Berg, 2008)	Focusing on problems and the past exacerbates problems	Identifying goals and solutions, and experiences of applying solutions, improves quality of life
Cognitive-behavioural therapy (Padesky & Mooney, 1990)	Thoughts, feelings, behaviours and biology interact; an unhelpful change in one leads to an unhelpful change in the others	Thoughts, feelings, behaviours and biology interact; a helpful change in one leads to a helpful change in the others
Narrative therapy (White, 2007)	A focus on unhelpful dominant stories leads to distress	Identifying or creating helpful stories can be freeing from distress
Capabilities approach (Nussbaum, 2009)	Limitations in what an individual is capable of doing and being adversely affects their quality of life.	Attaining and exercising freedom of choice to live a life valued by the individual improves quality of life

Appendix K
Worksheets and templates

Fundamentals of preparing for mentoring

This worksheet is a self-awareness resource to prepare you for the mentor role, covering two areas:

- Forming a vision of the mentor you want to become
- Reflecting on what you will bring to mentoring

Forming a vision of the mentor you want to become

A mentor role model

Forming a vision of the mentor you want to become may bring to mind memories of someone who was a significant figure in your development; someone who helped you to become who you are today. Did that person represent the type of mentor you want to become? If so, what qualities did they exhibit?

> Reflection #1 – A vision of the mentor I want to become:

Intentions

The Mentor's Charter is a reflective verse for mentors, containing examples of constructive intentions for the relational and developmental work of mentoring junior medical colleagues. You may recognise in the verse your own personal intentions.

In a spirit of goodwill, I choose to:
Value junior medical colleagues
Share with them my knowledge and experience
Connect them to resources
Encourage them on their way

Enable their achievements
Guide them in best practice and the ways of the profession
Demonstrate the value of reflection and lifelong learning
In doing so, I help them to be the best doctor they can be.

How do you intend to be a constructive influence on the mentee's development?

Reflection #2 – My constructive intentions as a mentor:

Style

A decision for you to make as a mentor will be the style of mentoring you offer, a way of engaging with mentees that feels natural and appropriate to you. In the book *Alpha Docs* (Munoz & Dale, 2014), Munoz reflects on his developmental experiences and the variety of ways in which senior doctors engaged with him during his training. Dr George was reassuring, providing guidance about what Munoz did well and could do better, and was always there as a safety net. Dr John let him find his own way, almost as though daring him to fail, and the closest he came to offering input was the question 'Are you sure?' Dr James' training style was described as executive: 'I trust you, give me the details that matter. What should you do?' Ultimately, Munoz concluded that maybe a little bit of fear is good for his learning. He credited Dr John's style with helping him to rely on himself, trust his judgment, push himself and handle pressure.

Reflection #3 – The style of mentoring I would like to offer:

Reflecting on what you will bring to mentoring

Attitudes and expectations

Your attitudes are ways of thinking and feeling about something, for example, a person, idea or situation, and relate to a tendency to respond positively or negatively. If you recognise in yourself a negative bias towards a mentee, consider where the bias has come from and how you will ensure your bias does not interfere with mentoring.

Attitude encompasses expectations you have of the mentee. You may have a baseline level of expectation that you apply to all of your mentoring partnerships, for example, a belief that mentees should not be 'spoon fed' and should figure things out for themselves as much as possible before approaching you for assistance. Recognising your expectations will enable you to readily discuss these with the mentee, which can help to avoid problems later.

Reflection #4 – My attitudes towards learners and novices, and my expectations of them:

Experiences

What experiences have you had as a doctor or mentor, that you could draw on for the benefit of the mentee? A related topic is how you approach new experiences. Do you shy away from the unfamiliar or do you take an open and willing approach to exploring new areas of practice, including research and other efforts to be innovative?

Reflection #5 – My past experiences as a doctor that may be of special interest to mentees are:

Reflection #6 – My past experiences as a mentor that will prepare me for future mentor roles

Reflection #7 – My willingness to explore new opportunities and experiences:

Strengths and limitations

What strengths do you bring to mentoring that could help the mentee in their efforts to develop? What are your areas of limitation? Recognising strengths and limitations enables you to put your strengths to work and manage your areas of limitation or vulnerability, for maximal effectiveness in your mentor role.

Reflection #8 – Areas of strength in my practice as a doctor and in my work assisting junior medical colleagues to develop:

Reflection #9 – Limitations in my practice as a doctor and in my work assisting junior medical colleagues to develop:

> Reflection #10 – The knowledge and or skills I need to develop further to be an effective mentor (*see* Appendix D, pp.205–7):

Availability

What amount of time can you set aside for mentoring, given your existing commitments? Are the commitments you are considering making to mentees achievable within your schedule?

> Reflection # 11 – My availability to help junior medical colleagues to develop:

Energy

Consider your energy reserves for engaging with mentees. How many mentoring partnerships could you be involved in, while preserving energy for existing commitments?

> Reflection # 12 – My energy for mentoring and the maximum number of mentees I could comfortably work with:

Mentee journal

This worksheet can be used by the mentee as a journal, to prepare for mentoring and to reflect on and record their progress during mentoring. The worksheet includes sample reflection questions and conversation starters, organised by area of the Australian Curriculum Framework for Junior Doctors (Confederation of Postgraduate Medical Education Councils, 2012).

Sample reflection questions & conversation starters	Date	Notes e.g. insights, decisions, plans, actions, results
Clinical management Patient assessment Safe patient care Acute and emergency care Patient management Skills and procedures In what area/s of practice do I feel most capable? In what area/s of practice do I feel unprepared? What can I do to address this? Based on feedback from my supervisors, are there areas of practice I could improve on? What is most challenging about my work? What is my attitude towards any medical mistakes that I make? How do I know that I am performing at the required level? To what extent do I pay attention to psychological and social aspects of my patients' illness? What has been the most significant professional experience for me so far this year? What resources and clinical guidelines are reliable for my day-to-day practice? Which hospital policies and procedures are relevant to my practice? How do I gauge the effectiveness of my clinical reasoning? What skills and procedures would I like more exposure to? What clinical problems and conditions would I like more exposure to? Other focus questions:		

Sample reflection questions & conversation starters	Date	Notes e.g. insights, decisions, plans, actions, results
Professionalism Doctor and society Professional behaviour Teaching, learning and supervision How do I see my role in the big picture of the health of my community? What contextual factors have an impact on how I am required to practice medicine? What are the limits to my role as doctor? What is my attitude towards asking for help when I need it? How do I actively sustain my resilience? What are the values that I want to enact in my practice? What practices do I adopt to ensure efficiency at work? What are some useful frameworks that can guide my work educating junior medical colleagues? Other focus questions:		
Communication Patient interaction Managing information Working in teams How do I manage patient expectations? Are there ways I try to avoid interacting with certain people, and why? What emotional reactions do I have to certain people and what are the likely origins of the reactions? Do I exhibit any behaviours that are preventing optimal care for patients? How do I show empathy with patients? How do I ensure appropriate clinician-patient boundaries are understood and maintained? How do I ensure that I behave lawfully in relation to confidential information? How do I structure information during case presentations and handover? How do I strive to work constructively with colleagues and patients I find difficult? Other focus questions:		

Mentoring agreement

This template can be used to formalise an agreement between you and the mentee.

INTENTIONAL MENTORING AGREEMENT

Between _____ (mentor) and _____ (mentee)

This agreement outlines aspects of the commitment we are making to mentoring, and the parameters we wish to set for the partnership and process for a time.

Why we will collaborate
Consider the purpose of mentoring e.g. for the mentee to acquire knowledge and skills, performance, and awareness and practise of values, and the mentee's initial goals

When we will collaborate
Consider the duration of the partnership, frequency of contact, and availability

What we will each contribute
Consider the responsibilities of the mentor and mentee

How we will keep in touch and work together
Consider methods of communication, and activities

What we will do if it doesn't go to plan
Consider the plan for resolving significant issues of concern within the partnership, that may arise during the course of mentoring

Signed: _____

[Mentor]   [Mentee]

Date:

Session checklists

Checklist for an initial partnership discussion

This checklist covers steps to take during an initial meeting with the mentee, as part of the empathic attachment stage of mentoring.

- ☐ Attempt to put the mentee at ease through open, genuine communication, considering verbal and non-verbal aspects of communication
- ☐ Identify initial goals for the mentee's development
- ☐ Identify the mentee's anticipated needs
- ☐ Discuss and reach a shared understanding of mentoring
- ☐ Decide whether to collaborate
- ☐ Discuss expectations, for example:
  - Confidentiality
  - Frequency of contact
  - Methods of communication
  - A contingency plan for conflict resolution
- ☐ Establish an agreement

Checklist for an initial goal-directed interaction

This checklist covers steps to take during an initial goal-directed interaction, as part of the active involvement stage of mentoring.

- ☐ Assist the mentee to identify their aspirational state of development and derive meaningful and relevant goals
- ☐ Invite the mentee to choose a goal for the session
- ☐ Identify the mentee's present situation relative to their goal
- ☐ Consider obstacles and options for the way forward
- ☐ Engage in activities that are likely to lead to goal achievement (based on the criteria of feasibility, plausibility and testability)
- ☐ Support, challenge and or facilitate as required
- ☐ Deliver brief interventions as required

Checklist for a follow-up session

This checklist covers steps to take during goal-directed interactions, as part of the active involvement stage of mentoring.

- [ ] Explore what the mentee did with the plans they made at the end of the last session, for the way forward. Did they follow through with their plans?
- [ ] Explore outcomes. What resulted from implementing the planned way forward? Did it change the mentee's reality to being closer to, or achieving, the goal?
- [ ] Clarify the goal for the current session. Is the goal the same or different?
- [ ] Identify obstacles and options to progress towards the goal
- [ ] Discuss the plan for the way forward

Checklist for a final session

This checklist covers steps to take as part of the felt separation stage of mentoring.

- [ ] Discuss the course of mentoring, highlighting memorable or significant moments
- [ ] Discuss the benefits and the effects of the mentoring, professionally and personally
- [ ] Discuss openness to maintain a level of contact in the future
- [ ] Identify actions that will allow you each to move forward separately and well

Mentee aspirational state of development

This worksheet can be used by the mentee to figure out their aspirational state of development.

Background

The mentee's aspirational state of development is central to developmental work. We define *aspirational state of development* as an ideal repertoire of knowing (a knowledge and skills base), doing (a set of performance behaviours) and being (awareness and practise of values) relevant to the mentee's job, career path and aspirations in the medical profession. The mentee's aspirational state of development serves as goal posts to aim for in developmental work and a benchmark for recognising development.

With the aspirational state of development goal posts decided for a time, goals may be set and pursued. Goals may relate to knowing (e.g. acquiring knowledge, skills and competencies), doing (e.g. accessing opportunities for participation and overcoming barriers to performance), or being (e.g. recognising and enacting values in practice). The mentor and mentee deliberately test out activities in service of goal achievement towards the mentee's aspirational state of development, and pay attention to results, continuing with what works and discontinuing what does not work. Collectively, goal achievement equates to progress towards or realisation of the aspirational state of development.

Exercise

To form an aspirational state of development, visualise and describe an ideal way of functioning in practice, based on the three dimensions of knowing, doing and being.

In the 'knowing' category, describe competencies relevant to work in a particular setting, at a level of seniority.
In the 'doing' category, describe essential tasks of practice.
In the 'being' category, describe values that will guide your practice, and qualities of practice.

Be as brief or as detailed as you like, and choose a format that suits you. Don't be too focused on capturing everything in words – this would be an impossible undertaking! Include enough detail to be able to derive meaningful and relevant goals.

Format 1

I want to become a doctor whose practice is characterised by:
- knowing (a dynamic knowledge and skills base) that includes –
- doing (a set of performance behaviours) that includes –
- being (aware of and practising values) that include –

Format 2

As a doctor I wish to:
- know and be able to –
- do –
- be –

Format 3

I wish to become a doctor who:
- can –
- does –
- is –

Format 4

As a doctor I wish to:
- have knowledge and skills that include –
- perform tasks that include –
- be guided by values that include –

Consider:
- a role model who exemplifies qualities you wish to develop
- a job description that outlines knowledge, skills and values required for your work
- the competency framework relevant to your training program

- mandatory and own choice aspects
- roles, level of performance, setting-specific considerations and regulations relevant to your practice
- weaknesses to address
- strengths to capitalise on
- the progress you wish to make by the end of a stage of training or a period of time.

Examples

"I want to become a doctor who:
- has knowledge and skills, as detailed in the Gastroenterology Advanced Training Curriculum and the Professional Qualities Curriculum
- performs tasks in the domains of practice described in the curricula, in ways that are appropriate for my local setting, at registrar level
- is resourceful, resilient and effective in making a difference to patients' experiences of their health."

"I want to become a gastroenterology registrar whose practice is characterised by:
- *Knowing* – I want to know the up to date literature around the common conditions I will see on a daily basis and know where to find the important information about things I will only come across rarely. I want to be able to integrate my knowledge and communication skills to deliver a patient-centred diagnostic and management plan.
- *Doing* – I want to deliver patient-centred diagnostic and management plans. I want to have a heavy focus on teaching and education of junior staff. I want to be involved in policy making in my specialty.
- *Being* – I want to be kind, compassionate and hard-working. I want to be humble, because it's the best thing for my patients. I want to be resilient, because it's necessary. I want my care to be holistic, and involve other experts when they're needed, but not waste their time when they're not needed. I want to consider not only the patient in front of me, but the broader healthcare environment when I'm making decisions."

Mentee reflection and goal setting

This worksheet can be used by the mentee to reflect on and set goals for mentoring, aligned with their aspirational state of development.

My aspirational state of development

Knowing – learning goals

Doing – performance goals

Being – values-related goals

Mentor reflections worksheet

Based on Gibbs' Reflective Cycle (Gibbs, 1988), this worksheet guides reflective practice of mentoring, after an episode of mentoring.

What types of activities took place in service of the mentee's goals?
What did you contribute to the interaction?
What did the mentee contribute to the interaction?
What thoughts and feelings arose in you during the interaction?
What aspects of the interaction did you perceive as positive and negative?
What was the significance of the interaction to you?
Would you adjust your practice, or do something differently in the next session? If so, what would that be?

Glossary

activities (process evaluation)	how inputs are transformed into actions in mentoring
activities, mentoring	conversations, actions and efforts within a mentoring partnership and process
aspirational state of development	an ideal repertoire of knowing, doing and being relevant to the mentee's job, career path and aspirations in the medical profession
attending (communication)	paying attention to all verbal and non-verbal cues in communication
bullying	repeated and unreasonable behaviour directed towards a worker or a group of workers that creates a risk to health and safety
CARE	commitment, accessibility, responsiveness, engagement
career path	direction for advancement in relation to career and preferred area of practice
challenge	strain-inducing resources benefiting the mentee in their development
competence	what the doctor has been trained to do
competency	an observable ability, skill or characteristic that can be measured and assessed with reliability and validity against a commonly agreed standard
deliberate practice	a type of practice that harnesses the adaptability of the human brain and body to create improvements in performance of a specific activity
developmental needs	resources benefiting an individual in their development
developmental outcomes (mentoring)	effects of mentoring on the mentee's development and adaptation
developmental work	work to foster development

doctor development	the doctor acquiring a repertoire of knowing (a dynamic knowledge and skills base), doing (a set of performance behaviours) and being (awareness and practise of values) relevant to their job and or career path in the medical profession.
facilitation	breakthrough-enabling resources benefiting the mentee in their development
following (communication)	following where the speaker is taking you
goal	the object of effort; a desired result
goals, mentoring	what the mentee wants to achieve through mentoring
goal-directed interaction	interaction that places one or more goals in focus, and uses the goal/s as a reference point for all collaborative efforts
I-Mentor with the Cycle of Caring	a visual representation of an intentional approach to the mentor's role
inputs (process evaluation)	resources invested in a process
job knowledge	a knowledge base explicitly taught in preparation for practice
MEAN	malice, ego, agenda and negativity
mediating mechanisms (performance)	the processes associated with executing and improving performance
mentee	the less experienced professional in a mentoring partnership
mentor (noun)	the more experienced professional in a mentoring partnership; an experienced professional with good intentions towards junior colleagues and the willingness to work with them and provide individually-relevant support, challenge and facilitation
mentor (verb)	to perform the role of mentor
mentor, intentional	a doctor who constructively and productively contributes to the development of junior medical colleagues
mentoring, intentional	a mentoring methodology with a system of principles and practices; the pursuit of developmental outcomes that are meaningful to the mentee, at the centre of a constructive partnership and a productive process
Model of Intentional Mentoring	a visual representation of the course of a mentoring partnership and process

needs, comparative	need revealed through the services required by a similar population
needs, expressed	need inferred through the uptake of services
needs, felt	what the mentee says they need
needs, normative	what a credible authority says the mentee needs
outcome evaluation	determination of the outcomes and effects of a process
outcomes	intended and unintended effects
outputs (process evaluation)	the products of mentoring; the signs of the mentor and mentee's level of engagement
partnership (mentoring)	an alliance for doctor development
performance	what the doctor actually does from day to day
process (mentoring)	a series of actions in service of the mentee's development
process evaluation	a description of inputs, activities and outputs
reflecting (communication)	confirming understanding of a message through reflecting, paraphrasing and summarising
relational work	work to build relationship
session (mentoring)	an episode of mentoring
strategy	a plan of action designed to achieve an aim
support	strengthening resources benefiting the mentee in their development
tacit knowledge	knowledge that is learned on the job via experience, and is not explicitly taught
toolkit, intentional mentor's	ten tools to enable a mentor to be a constructive and productive contributor to the mentee's development
values	standards or principles considered valuable or important in life

References

ABIM Foundation, ACP–ASIM Foundation, & European Federation of Internal Medicine. (2002). Medical professionalism in the new Millennium: A physician charter, 5 February 2002. *Annals of Internal Medicine, 136*(3), 243-246. http://dx.doi.org/10.7326/0003

Ahern, S. F., Morley, P. T., & McColl, G. J. (2016). Governing the reform of the medical internship. *Medical Journal of Australia, 204*(10), 374-375. http://dx.doi.org/10.5694/mja15.01326

Aspen Institute. Roundtable on Comprehensive Community Initiatives for Children and Families. (1997). *Voices from the field: Learning from the early work of comprehensive community initiatives*. Washington, DC: Aspen Institute.

Australian Health Practitioner Regulation Agency. (2016). *Mandatory reporting*. Retrieved September 7, 2016 from AHPRA website: http://www.ahpra.gov.au/Notifications/Make-a-complaint/Mandatory-notifications.aspx

Australian Medical Association. (2010). *Competency-based training in medical education, 2010*. Retrieved May 10 2016, from https://ama.com.au/position-statement/competency-based-training-medical-education-2010

Australian Medical Council. (2014). *Intern training – Intern outcome statements*. Retrieved May 15, 2016 from Medical Board of Australia website: http://www.medicalboard.gov.au/Registration/Interns/Guidelines-resources-tools.aspx

Australian Public Health Nutrition Academic Collaboration. (2005). *A mentoring framework for public health nutrition workforce development.* Wollongong: APHNAC. Retrieved from APHNAC website http://www.voced.edu.au/content/ngv%3A46702

Berg, K. & Latin, R. (2007). *Essentials of research methods in health, physical education, exercise science and recreation* (3rd ed.). Sydney: Lippincott, Williams & Wilkins.

beyondblue (2013). *National mental health survey of doctors and medical students*. Retrieved from http://www.beyondblue.org.au/dmhp

Bozeman, B., & Feeney, M. K. (2007). Toward a useful theory of mentoring: A conceptual analysis and critique. *Administration & Society, 39*(6), 719-739. http://dx.doi.org/10.1177/0095399707304119

Bradshaw J. (1972). A taxonomy of social need. In G. McLachlan (Ed.), *Problems and progress in medical care* (p. 69). Oxford: Oxford University Press. Retrieved from http://www.york.ac.uk/inst/spru/pubs/pdf/JRB.pdf

Broadwell, M.M. (1969). Teaching for learning (XVI). *The Gospel Guardian, 20*(41), 1-3a. Retrieved from http://www.wordsfitlyspoken.org/gospel_guardian/v20/v20n41p1-3a.html

Cantillon, P., & Sargeant, J. (2008). Giving feedback in clinical settings. *BMJ (Clinical Research Ed.), 337*, a1961. http://dx.doi.org/10.1136/bmj.a1961

Centers for Disease Control and Prevention. (2008). *Introduction to process evaluation in tobacco use prevention and control*. Atlanta, GA: U.S. Dept. of Health & Human Services, CDC. Retrieved from http://www.cdc.gov/tobacco/publications/index.htm

Cervero, R. M., & Gaines, J. K. (2015). The impact of CME on physician performance and patient health outcomes: An updated synthesis of systematic reviews. *Journal of Continuing Education in the Health Professions, 35*(2), 131-138. http://dx.doi.org/10.1002/chp.21290

Cianciolo, A. T., Matthew, C., Sternberg, R. J., & Wagner, R. K. (2006). Tacit knowledge, practical intelligence, and expertise. In K. A. Ericsson, N. Charness, P. J. Feltovich & R. R. Hoffman (Eds.), *The Cambridge handbook of expertise and expert performance* (pp. 613-632). New York: Cambridge University Press.

Clancey, W. J. (2006). Observation of work practices in natural settings. In K. A. Ericsson, N. Charness, P. J. Feltovich & R. R. Hoffman (Eds.), *The Cambridge handbook of expertise and expert performance* (pp. 127-145). New York: Cambridge University Press.

Colbert, C. Y., Graham, L., West, C., White, B. A., Arroliga, A. C., Myers, J. D., . . . Clark, J. (2015). Teaching metacognitive skills: Helping your physician trainees in the quest to 'know what they don't know'. *The American Journal of Medicine, 128*(3), 318-324. http://dx.doi.org/10.1016/j.amjmed.2014.11.001

Collins, A. (2005). Cognitive apprenticeship. In: R. K. Sawyer (Ed.), *The Cambridge handbook of the learning sciences* (pp. 47-60). Cambridge, UK: Cambridge University Press.

Confederation of Postgraduate Medical Education Councils. (2012). *Australian curriculum framework for junior doctors*. Retrieved May 17, 2016 from http://curriculum.cpmec.org.au/index.cfm

Cooperrider, D.L., Whitney, D., & Stavros, J.M. (2008). *Appreciative enquiry handbook: For leaders of change* (2nd ed.). Brunswick, OH: Crown Custom Publishing.

Cruess, R. L., Cruess, S. R., & Steinert, Y. (2016). Amending Miller's Pyramid to include professional identity formation. *Academic Medicine: Journal of the Association of American Medical Colleges, 91*(2), 180-185. http://dx.doi.org/10.1097/ACM.0000000000000913

Cutlip, S. M., & Center, A. H. (1952). *Effective public relations: pathways to public favour.* New York: Prentice-Hall.

De Jong, P., & Berg, I. K. (2008). *Interviewing for solutions* (3rd ed.). Belmont, CA: Thomson Higher Education.

Doherty, C. (2004). Introducing mentoring to doctors: Challenging the sink or swim culture. *Development and Learning in Organizations: An International Journal, 18*(1), 6-8. Retrieved from http://search.ebscohost.com/login.aspx?direct=true&AuthType=ip,athens&db=edb&AN=70440038&site=eds-live

Dominguez, N., & Hager, M. (2013). Mentoring frameworks: synthesis and critique. *International Journal of Mentoring and Coaching in Education, 2*(3), 171-188. http://dx.doi.org/10.1108/IJMCE-03-2013-0014

Doran, G. T. (1981). There's a S.M.A.R.T. way to write management's goals and objectives. *Management Review, 70*(11), 35-36.

Dunning, D., Johnson, K., Ehrlinger, J. & Kruger, J. (2003). Why people fail to recognize their own incompetence, *Current Directions in Psychological Science, 12*(3), 83-87. http://dx.doi.org/10.1111/1467-8721.01235

Eby, L. T. (2012). Workplace mentoring: Past, present, and future perspectives. In S. W. J. Kozlowski (Ed.), *The Oxford handbook of organizational psychology, 1,* 615-642. New York: Oxford University Press.

Egan, G. (2002). *The skilled helper: A problem-management and opportunity-development approach to helping* (7th ed.). Pacific Grove, CA: Brooks/Cole Publishing.

Eichbaum, Q. G. (2014). Thinking about thinking and emotion: The metacognitive approach to the medical humanities that integrates the humanities with the basic and clinical sciences. *The Permanente Journal, 18(*4), 64-75. http://dx.doi.org/10.7812/TPP/14-027

Ende, J. (1983). Feedback in clinical medical education. JAMA: *The Journal of the American Medical Association, 250*(6), 777-781. http://dx.doi.org/10.1001/jama.1983.03340060055026.

Engeström, Y. (1999). Expansive visibilization of work: An activity-theoretical perspective. *Computer Supported Cooperative Work* (CSCW), 8(1), 63-93. http://dx.doi.org/10.1023/A:1008648532192

Epstein, R.M. & Krasner, M.S. (2013). Physician resilience: What it means, why it matters, and how to promote it. *Academic Medicine: Journal of the Association of American Medical Colleges, 88*(3), 301-303. http://dx.doi.org/10.1097/ACM.0b013e318280cff0

Ericsson, K. A. (2004). Deliberate practice and the acquisition and maintenance of expert performance in medicine and related domains. *Academic Medicine: Journal of the Association of American Medical Colleges, 79*(10), S70-S81.

Ericsson, K. A. (2006). The influence of experience and deliberate practice on the development of superior expert performance. In K. A. Ericsson, N. Charness, P. J. Feltovich & R. R. Hoffman (Eds.), *The Cambridge handbook of expertise and expert performance* (pp. 683-703). New York: Cambridge University Press.

Ericsson, K. A. (2007). Deliberate practice and the modifiability of body and mind: Toward a science of the structure and acquisition of expert and elite performance. *International Journal of Sport Psychology, 38(*1), 4-34. Retrieved from http://search.ebscohost.com/login.aspx?direct=true&AuthType=ip,athens&db=psyh&AN=2007-06716-002&site=eds-live

Ericsson, K. A. (2009). *Development of professional expertise: Toward measurement of expert performance and design of optimal learning environments.* New York: Cambridge University Press.

Ericsson, K. A. (2015). Acquisition and maintenance of medical expertise: A perspective from the expert-performance approach with deliberate practice. *Academic Medicine: Journal of the Association of American Medical Colleges, 90*(11), 1471-1486. http://dx.doi.org/10.1097/ACM.0000000000000939

Ericsson, K. A. & Pool, R. (2016). *Peak: Secrets from the new science of expertise*. New York: Houghton Mifflin Harcourt Publishing Company.

Ethics Unwrapped (2016). *Giving voice to values* [DVD series]. Austin: University of Texas at Austin. Retrieved from http://ethicsunwrapped.utexas.edu/video/introduction-to-giving-voice-to-values

Feltovich, P. J., Prietula, M. J., & Ericsson, K. A. (2006). Studies of expertise from psychological perspectives. In K. A. Ericsson, N. Charness, P. J. Feltovich & R. R. Hoffman (Eds.), *The Cambridge handbook of expertise and expert performance* (pp. 41-67). New York: Cambridge University Press.

Flavell, J. (1987). Speculations about the nature and development of metacognition. In F.E. Weinert & R.H. Kluwe (Eds.), *Metacognition, motivation and understanding* (pp. 21-29). Hillsdale, NJ: Lawrence Erlbaum Associates.

Frank J.R., Snell L.S., Sherbino J., et al. (2014). *Draft CanMEDS 2015 Milestones Guide – September 2014*. Ottawa: Royal College of Physicians and Surgeons of Canada. Retrieved from Royal College website: http://www.royalcollege.ca/portal/page/portal/rc/common/documents/canmeds/framework/canmeds_milestone_guide_sept2014_e.pdf

Frank, J.R., Snell, L., & Sherbino, J. (Eds.) (2015). *CanMEDS 2015 physician competency framework*. Ottawa: Royal College of Physicians and Surgeons of Canada. Retrieved from Royal College website: http://www.royalcollege.ca/portal/page/portal/rc/common/documents/canmeds/framework/canmeds_full_framework_e.pdf

Gabel, S. (2011). Addressing demoralization in clinical staff: A true test of leadership. *Journal of Nervous and Mental Disease*, *199*(11):892–895. http://dx.doi.org/10.1097/NMD.0b013e3182349e79

Gabel, S. (2011). Ethics and values in clinical practice: Whom do they help? *Mayo Clinic Proceedings*, *86*(5), 421-424. http://dx.doi.org/10.4065/mcp.2010.0781

Gabel, S. (2013). Demoralization in health professional practice: development, amelioration, and implications for continuing education. *The Journal of Continuing Education in the Health Professions, 33*(2), 118-126. http://dx.doi.org/10.1002/chp.21175

Gibbs, G. (1988). *Learning by doing: A guide to teaching and learning methods*. Oxford: Further Education Unit.

Gilbert, T. F. (1978). *Human competence: Engineering worthy performance*. New York: McGraw-Hill.

Godlee, F. (2008). Understanding the role of the doctor. BMJ: *British Medical Journal, 337*(7684), 1425-1426. http://dx.doi.org/10.1136/bmj.a3035

Hafferty, F.W. & Franks, R. (1994). The hidden curriculum, ethics teaching, and the structure of medical education. *Academic Medicine: Journal of the Association of American Medical Colleges, 69*(11), 861-871. http://dx.doi.org/10.1136/bmj.329.7469.770

Hafferty, F.W. (2006). Professionalism – The next wave. *New England Journal of Medicine, 355* (20), 2151-2152. http://dx.doi.org/10.1056/NEJMe068217

Hagerty, B. (1986). A second look at mentors. *Nursing Outlook, 34*(1), 16-19, 24.

Harris, R. (2007). *The happiness trap: Stop struggling, start living*. Wollombi, NSW: Exisle Publishing.

Haughey, D. (2014, December 13). A brief history of SMART goals [Blog post]. Retrieved from https://www.projectsmart.co.uk/brief-history-of-smart-goals.php

Hayes, S., & Smith, S. (2005). *Get out of your mind and into your life: The new acceptance and commitment therapy*. Oaklands, CA: New Harbinger Publications.

Jensen, P.M., Trollope-Kumar, K., Waters, H. & Everson, J. (2008). Building physician resilience. *Canadian Family Physician, 54*(5), 722-729. Retrieved from http://www.cfp.ca/content/54/5/722.full.pdf+html

Johnson, S. (2008). *Hold me tight: Seven conversations for a lifetime of love*. Boston: Little, Brown & Co.

Johnson, W. B. (2002). The intentional mentor: strategies and guidelines for the practice of mentoring. *Professional Psychology: Research and Practice, 33*(1), 88-96. http://dx.doi.org/10.1037/0735-7028.33.1.88

Jones, V. (2014, August 3). What is the most important trait in a doctor? [Blog post]. Retrieved from http://www.kevinmd.com/blog/2014/08/important-trait-doctor.html

Kirkpatrick, D. L. (1967). Evaluation of training. In R.L. Craig & L.R. Bittel (Eds.), *Training and development handbook* (pp. 87–112). New York: McGraw Hill.

Knowles, M. (1984). *The adult learner: A neglected species* (3rd ed.). Houston, TX: Gulf Publishing.

Kotzman, A. (1989). *Listen to me, listen to you*. Ringwood, Vic: Penguin Books Australia.

Lake, F.R. & Hamdorf, J.M. (2004). Teaching on the run tips 5: Teaching a skill. *Medical Journal of Australia, 181*(6): 327-328. Retrieved from http://www.rdi.uwa.edu.au/__data/assets/pdf_file/0006/99348/tip5.pdf

Lake, F.R., & Ryan, G. (2004). Teaching on the run tips 3: Planning a teaching episode. *Medical Journal of Australia*, *180*(12), 643-644.

Lave, J., & Wenger, E. (1991) *Situated learning: Legitimate peripheral participation*. Cambridge: Cambridge University Press.

Leach, D.C. (2002). Competence is a habit. *Journal of the American Medical Association, 287*, 243–44. http://dx.doi.org/10.1001/jama.287.2.243

Leach, D.C. (2004). Professionalism: The formation of physicians. *The American Journal of Bioethics, 4*(2), 11-12. http://dx.doi.org/10.1162/152651604323097619

Leape, L., Shore, M., & Dienstag, J. L. (2013). In reply to Alexander et al. [letter]. *Academic Medicine: Journal of the Association of American Medical Colleges, 88*(6), 741-744. http://dx.doi.org/10.1097/ACM.0b013e318290b63c

Lehmann, A. C., & Gruber, H. (2006). Music. In K. A. Ericsson, N. Charness, P. J. Feltovich & R. R. Hoffman (Eds.), *The Cambridge handbook of expertise and expert performance* (pp. 457-470). New York: Cambridge University Press.

Leiter, M. P., Frank, E., & Matheson, T. J. (2009). Demands, values, and burnout: Relevance for physicians. *Canadian Family Physician, 55*(12):1224–1225.e1–6. Retrieved from http://www.cfp.ca/content/55/12/1224.short

MacDonald, G., Starr, G., Schooley, M., Yee, S.L., Klimowski, K., & Turner, K. (2001). *Introduction to program evaluation for comprehensive tobacco control programs*. Retrieved from Centers for Disease Control and Prevention website: http://www.cdc.gov/tobacco/stateandcommunity/tobacco_control_programs/surveillance_evaluation/evaluation_manual/pdfs/evaluation.pdf

Maté, G. (2003). *When the body says no: Exploring the stress-disease connection*. New Jersey: John Wiley & Sons, Inc.

McDaniel Jr, R. R., Lanham, H. J., & Anderson, R. A. (2009). Implications of complex adaptive systems theory for the design of research on health care organizations. *Health Care Management Review, 34*(2), 191-199. http://dx.doi.org/10.1097/HMR.0b013e31819c8b38

Medical Board of Australia. (2014). *Good medical practice: A code of conduct for doctors in Australia.* Retrieved May 12, 2016 from http://www.medicalboard.gov.au/Codes-Guidelines-Policies/Code-of-conduct.aspx

Mehrabian, A. (1981). *Silent messages: Implicit communication of emotions and attitudes* (2nd ed.). Belmont, CA: Wadsworth.

Miller, G.E. (1990). The assessment of clinical skills/competence/performance. *Academic Medicine: Journal of the Association of American Medical Colleges, 65*(9), S63-67. Retrieved from http://journals.lww.com/academicmedicine/Abstract/1990/09000/The_assessment_of_clinical.45.aspx

Munoz, D. & Dale, J.M. (2014). *Alpha docs: The making of a cardiologist.* New York: Random House.

Murphy, D.J., Guthrie, B., Sullivan, F.M., Mercer, S.W., Russell, A., & Bruce, D.A. (2012). Insightful practice: A reliable measure for medical revalidation. *BMJ Quality and Safety, 21*(8):649-656. http://dx.doi.org/10.1136/bmjqs-2011-000429

Musselman, L. J., MacRae, H. M., Reznick, R. K., & Lingard, L. A. (2005). 'You learn better under the gun': Intimidation and harassment in surgical education. *Medical Education, 39*(9), 926-934. http://dx.doi.org/10.1111/j.1365-2929.2005.02247.x

Neher, J. O., & Stevens, N. G. (2003). The one-minute preceptor: shaping the teaching conversation. *Family Medicine, 35*(6), 391-393. Retrieved from http://www.stfm.org/Portals/49/Documents/FMPDF/FamilyMedicineVol35Issue6Neher391.pdf

Neher, J.O., Gordon, K.C., Meyer, B., & Stevens, N. (1992). A five-step microskills model of clinical teaching. *Journal of the American Board of Family Practice, 5*(4), 419-24. http://dx.doi.org/10.3122/jabfm.5.4.419

Norman, G., Eva, K., Brooks, L., & Hamstra, S. (2006). Expertise in medicine and surgery. In K. A. Ericsson, N. Charness, P. J. Feltovich & R. R. Hoffman (Eds.), *The Cambridge handbook of expertise and expert performance* (pp. 339-353). New York: Cambridge University Press.

Nussbaum, M. C. (2009). Creating capabilities: The human development approach and its implementation. *Hypatia: A Journal of Feminist Philosophy, 24*(3), 211-215. http://dx.doi.org/10.1111/j.1527-2001.2009.01052_1.x

Padesky, C. A., & Mooney, K. A. (1990). Presenting the cognitive model to clients. *International Cognitive Therapy Newsletter, 6*(1), 13-14.

Pangaro, L. (1999). A new vocabulary and other innovations for improving descriptive in-training evaluation. *Academic Medicine: Journal of the Association of American Medical Colleges, 74*(11), 1203-1207. http://dx.doi.org/10.1097/00001888-199911000-00012

Phillips, S. P., & Clarke, M. (2012). More than an education: The hidden curriculum, professional attitudes and career choice. *Medical Education, 46*(9), 887-893. http://dx.doi.org/10.1111/j.1365-2923.2012.04316.x

Pintrich, P. R. (2002). The role of metacognitive knowledge in learning, teaching, and assessing. *Theory into Practice, 41*(4), 219-225. http://dx.doi.org/10.1207/s15430421tip4104_3

Quirk, M. (2006). *Intuition and metacognition in medical education: Keys to developing expertise.* New York: Springer.

Rabow, M. W., Remen, R. N., Parmelee, D. X., & Inui, T. S. (2010). Professional formation: Extending medicine's lineage of service into the next century. *Academic Medicine: Journal of the Association of American Medical Colleges, 85*(2), 310-317. http://dx.doi.org/10.1097/ACM.0b013e3181c887f7

Ramage, J. D., Bean, J. C., & Johnson, J. (2012). *Writing arguments; a rhetoric with readings* (9th ed.). Boston: Pearson.

Rautio, A., Sunnari, V., Nuutinen, M., & Laitala, M. (2005). Mistreatment of university students most common during medical studies. *BMC Medical Education, 5*, 36. http://dx.doi.org/10.1186/1472-6920-5-36

Rethans, J., Norcini, J. J., Barón-Maldonado, M., Blackmore, D., Jolly, B. C., LaDuca, T., . . . Southgate, L. H. (2002). The relationship between competence and performance: Implications for assessing practice performance. *Medical Education, 36*(10), 901-909. http://dx.doi.org/10.1046/j.1365-2923.2002.01316.x

Roberts, A. (1999). The origins of the term mentor. *History of Education Society Bulletin, 64*, 313-329.

Roberts, A. (2000). Mentoring revisited: A phenomenological reading of the literature, *Mentoring & Tutoring: Partnership in Learning, 8*(2), 145-170. http://dx.doi.org/10.1080/713685524

Robinson, A. (1993). *What smart students know: Maximum grades, optimum learning, minimum time.* New York: Crown Trade Paperbacks.

Rothschild, B., & Rand, M.L. (2006). *Help for the helper: The psychophysiology of compassion fatigue and vicarious trauma*. New York: Norton.

Royal Australasian College of Physicians. (2010). *Supporting physicians' professionalism and performance: A literature review.* Retrieved May 13, 2016 from https://www.racp.edu.au/docs/default-source/default-document-library/sppp-literature-review.pdf?sfvrsn=2

Royal Australasian College of Surgeons (2016). *JDocs framework: A guide for junior doctors* (Ver. 2). Melbourne: RACS. Retrieved May 10, 2016 from RACS website http://jdocs.surgeons.org/sites/jdocs/files/jdocs_framework_v6_final%20artwork.pdf

Royal Australasian College of Surgeons, Expert Advisory Group on Discrimination, Bullying and Sexual Harassment Advising the Royal Australasian College of Surgeons. (2015). *Report to the Royal Australasian College of Surgeons, 28 September 2015.* Retrieved from RACS website: https://www.surgeons.org/media/22086656/EAG-Report-to-RACS-FINAL-28-September-2015-.pdf

Royal College of Physicians of London. (2005). *Doctors in society: Medical professionalism in a changing world: Report of a working party, December 2005.* London: Royal College of Physicians of London. Retrieved from http://shop.rcplondon.ac.uk/products/doctors-in-society-medical-professionalism-in-a-changing-world?variant=6337443013

Rudolph, J. W., Simon, R., Raemer, D. B., & Eppich, W. J. (2008). Debriefing as formative assessment: Closing performance gaps in medical education. *Academic Emergency Medicine: Official Journal of the Society for Academic Emergency Medicine, 15*(11), 1010-1016. http://dx.doi.org/10.1111/j.1553-2712.2008.00248.x

Rudolph, J. W., Simon, R., Rivard, P., Dufresne, R. L., & Raemer, D. B. (2007). Debriefing with good judgment: Combining rigorous feedback with genuine inquiry. *Anesthesiology Clinics, 25*, 361-376. http://dx.doi.org/10.1016/j.anclin.2007.03.007

Ryan, C. A. (2010). Reflective inquiry in the medical profession. In N. Lyons (Ed.) *Handbook of reflection and reflective inquiry: Mapping a way of knowing for professional reflective inquiry* (pp. 101-130). New York: Springer. http://dx.doi.org/10.1007/978-0-387-85744-2_6

Salvador, D. & Collings, R. (2014). *Mentoring doctors: how to design and implement a junior doctor mentoring program.* Douglas, Qld: The Authors.

Schön, D. A. (1983). *The reflective practitioner: How professionals think in action*. New York: Basic Books.

Schön, D. A. (1987). *Educating the reflective practitioner: Toward a new design for teaching and learning in the professions*. San Francisco, CA: Jossey-Bass Publishers.

Scott, K. M., Caldwell, P. H., Barnes, E. H., & Barrett, J. (2015). 'Teaching by humiliation' and mistreatment of medical students in clinical rotations: A pilot study. *Medical Journal of Australia, 203*(4), 181-185. http://dx.doi.org/doi: 10.5694/mja15.00189

Siegel, D.J. (2010). *Mindsight: A new science of personal transformation*. New York: Bantam Books.

Skovholt, T. M. (2005). The cycle of caring: A model of expertise in the helping professions. *Journal of Mental Health Counseling, 27*(1), 82-93. Retrieved from http://search.ebscohost.com/login.aspx?direct=true&AuthType=ip,athens&db=pbh&AN=15674303&site=eds-live

Skovholt, T.M. & Trotter-Mathison, M. (2016). *The resilient practitioner: Burnout and compassion fatigue prevention and self-care strategies for the helping professions* (3rd ed.). New York: Routledge.

Souba W.W. (2011). The being of leadership. *Philosophy, Ethics and Humanities in Medicine, 6*, 5. http://dx.doi.org/10.1186/1747-5341-6-5

Spencer, L. 1989. *Winning through participation: Meeting the challenge of corporate change with the technology of participation*. Dubuque: Kendall Hunt Publishing.

Stephen, A., Oxley, J., & Fleming, W.G. (2008). Mentoring for NHS doctors: Perceived benefits across the personal-professional interface, *Journal of the Royal Society of Medicine, 101*(11), 552-557. http://dx.doi.org/10.1258/jrsm.2008.080153

Stratton-Berkessel, R. (2010). *Appreciative enquiry for collaborative solutions.* San Francisco, CA: Pfeiffer.

Tanner, K. D. (2012). Promoting student metacognition. *CBE Life Sciences Education, 11*(2), 113-120. http://dx.doi.org/10.1187/cbe.12-03-0033

Turner, G. W., & Turner, B. (Eds.) (1989). *The Australian Oxford paperback dictionary* (1st Australian ed). Melbourne: Oxford University Press.

Vogt E., Brown, J., & Isaacs, D. (2003). *The art of powerful questions: Catalyzing insight, innovation and action.* Waltham, MA: Whole Systems Associates. Retrieved from SPARC BC website https://www.principals.ca/documents/powerful_questions_article_ (World_Cafe_Website).pdf

Weisberg, R. W. (2006). Modes of expertise in creative thinking: Evidence from case studies. In K. A. Ericsson, N. Charness, P. J. Feltovich, & R. R. Hoffman (Eds.), *The Cambridge handbook of expertise and expert performance* (pp. 761-787). New York: Cambridge University Press.

Wenger-Trayner, E., & Wenger-Trayner, B. (2015). *Introduction to communities of practice: A brief overview of the concept and its uses.* Retrieved from http://wenger-trayner.com/wp-content/uploads/2015/04/07-Brief-introduction-to-communities-of-practice.pdf

White, M. (2007). *Maps of narrative practice.* New York: WW Norton & Co.

Whitmore, J. (2009). *Coaching for performance: GROWing human potential and purpose: The principles and practice of coaching and leadership* (4th ed.). London: Nicholas Brealey Publishing.

Wilson, A. & Feyer, A.M. (2015). *Review of medical intern training final report, Australian Health Ministers' Advisory Council.* Adelaide: COAG Health Council. Retrieved from COAG Health Council website http://www.coaghealthcouncil.gov.au/ Portals/0/Review%20of%20Medical%20Intern%20Training%20Final%20Report%20 publication%20version.pdf

Annotated Bibliography

This list highlights ten articles from the Reference section, that were most significant in shaping our thoughts about mentoring and the mentor role, and inspiring the ideas in this book. We highly recommend these articles to readers who wish to learn more about mentoring and the mentor role.

Bozeman, B., & Feeney, M. K. (2007). Toward a useful theory of mentoring: A conceptual analysis and critique. *Administration & Society, 39*(6), 719-739. http://dx.doi.org/10.1177/0095399707304119
Mentoring is commonplace, yet fundamental conceptual and theoretical issues have been skirted in the research and in the literature. "If everything is mentoring, nothing is", remark Bozeman and Feeney. They state the need for conceptual development of mentoring, make suggestions for conceptual boundaries, and offer a definition of mentoring. *see* **The elusive concept of mentoring** (Chapter 1, p.3).

Cruess, R. L., Cruess, S. R., & Steinert, Y. (2016). Amending Miller's pyramid to include professional identity formation. *Academic Medicine: Journal of the Association of American Medical Colleges, 91*(2), 180-185. http://dx.doi.org/10.1097/ACM.0000000000000913
Miller's pyramid, a representation of competence and performance in medicine, emphasises what a doctor knows and does as a doctor. Cruess, Cruess and Steinert suggest that Miller's pyramid requires an additional level to emphasize the significance of who a doctor is, and presents an argument for the source of professionalism being professional identity, with an emphasis on values. *see* **Knowing, doing and being in the medical profession** (Chapter 2, p.32).

Doherty, C. (2004). Introducing mentoring to doctors: Challenging the sink or swim culture. *Development & Learning in Organizations: An International Journal, 18*(1), 6-8. Retrieved from http://search.ebscohost.com/login.aspx?direct=true&AuthType=ip,athens&db=edb&AN=70440038&site=eds-live
Doherty explains why mentoring is important in the field of medicine. New medical graduates are often thrown in the deep end and left to their own devices to survive the challenging conditions of the medical profession. Mentoring provides an alternative

to the sink or swim culture. Through mentoring, doctors have a safe space to talk with colleagues about themselves and their experiences. Doherty also explains how mentoring and medical practice are distinct, with a comparison that reveals several distinctions and gives definition to the concept of mentoring. *see* **The mentor role is not the doctor role** (Chapter 4, p.49).

Dominguez, N., & Hager, M. (2013). Mentoring frameworks: synthesis and critique. *International Journal of Mentoring and Coaching in Education, 2*(3), 171-188. Retrieved from http://search.ebscohost.com/login.aspx?direct=true&AuthType=ip,athens&db= edo&AN=ejs35132232&site=eds-live
Dominguez and Hager contribute a comprehensive summary of theoretical frameworks for understanding mentoring within three categories: developmental (transitions), learning and social. Many professionals and organisations proceed with mentoring without having a theory underpinning mentoring or explaining the purpose of mentoring. Dominguez and Hager's contribution helps professionals and organisations to design programs and partnerships using theory to guide. They also provide suggestions for mentoring scholarship. Although their recommendations are for universities, these also have relevance for medicine. *see* **Intentional mentoring** (Chapter 1, p.5).

Eby, L. T. (2012). Workplace mentoring: Past, present, and future perspectives. In S. W. J. Kozlowski (Ed.), *The Oxford handbook of organizational psychology*, 1, 615-642. New York, NY, US: Oxford University Press.
Eby reviews existing research on mentoring from the perspectives of both the mentor and the mentee (called the protégé) in one on one hierarchical relationships. She provides a developmental perspective of mentoring, and through this lens reveals factors associated with initiation, maturation and decline of mentoring relationships, as well as contextual factors influencing mentoring, particularly the organisational setting. Eby explains that understanding mentoring requires an understanding of the full range of relational experiences that can occur in mentoring, both positive and negative. She reminds us that it is normal for all close relationships to have positive and negative aspects. Finally, Eby outlines methodological issues and future possibilities in the study of mentoring. *see* **Intentional mentoring** (Chapter 1, p.5) and **How to use the tool** (Chapter 6, p.75).

Gabel, S. (2013). Demoralization in health professional practice: development, amelioration, and implications for continuing education. *The Journal of Continuing Education in the Health Professions, 33*(2), 118-126. http://dx.doi.org/10.1002/chp.21175

Demoralization and burnout are real issues in health professions and all health professionals are at risk. An explanation for demoralization is values-related conflicts. Gabel presents ideas for what individuals and organisations can do to prevent demoralization and change conditions of practice. *see* **Why is intentional mentoring useful in the field of medicine?** (Chapter 1, p.17) and **How to use the tool** (Chapter 10, p.105).

Johnson, W. B. (2002). The intentional mentor: strategies and guidelines for the practice of mentoring. *Professional Psychology: Research and Practice 33*(1), 88-96. Retrieved from http://search.ebscohost.com/login.aspx?direct=true&AuthType=ip,athens&db=edsgao&AN=edsgcl.83032416&site=eds-live
Written from the perspective of a psychologist working in the field of psychology, Johnson states that psychologists are increasingly called upon to mentor, and few receive training in the science and art of mentoring. The same could be said of doctors in the field of medicine. Johnson encourages a transition in the profession's concept of mentoring, from a secondary duty to an intentional activity, requiring a framework that involves intentional preparation and careful application. *see* **Intentional mentoring** (Chapter 1, p.5).

Rabow, M. W., Remen, R. N., Parmelee, D. X., & Inui, T. S. (2010). Professional formation: Extending medicine's lineage of service into the next century. *Academic Medicine: Journal of the Association of American Medical Colleges, 85*(2), 310-317. http://dx.doi.org/10.1097/ACM.0b013e3181c887f7
Rabow, Remen, Parmelee and Inui explain why values matter in medical practice, how practising science and humanism values in a balanced way makes scientific medical practice humanly relevant, and how students and doctors can be assisted to tether to their personal and professional values through professional formation. *see* ***Introduction, p.xix*** and **Why is intentional mentoring useful in the field of medicine?** (Chapter 1, pp.16–17).

Roberts, A. (1999). The origins of the term mentor. *History of Education Society Bulletin 64*, 313-329.
The literary origins of the word mentor, in Homer's epic poem Odyssey, do not resolve difficulties in the definitional clarity of the term mentor and the action mentoring. Roberts argues that "the extrapolation of the attributes of Homer's Mentor into modern day mentoring is illusory". Homer did not endow the character Mentor with qualities analogous with the current use of the term mentor, as one who counsels, guides, nurtures and advises. In the 18th century, Fénelon re-created the character Mentor in Les Aventures de Télémaque, and it is Fénelon's Mentor, not Homer's Mentor, who resembles the way we think of a mentor today. *see* **The elusive concept of mentoring** (Chapter 1, p.3).

Skovholt, T. M. (2005). The Cycle of Caring: A Model of Expertise in the Helping Professions. *Journal of Mental Health Counseling, 27*(1), 82-93. Retrieved from http://search.ebscohost.com/login.aspx?direct=true&AuthType=ip,athens&db=pbh&AN=15674303&site=eds-live

Shovholt's original Cycle of Caring is a model of expertise that guides helping professionals through three stages of helping: empathic attachment, active involvement and felt separation, for effective, sustainable practice. *see* **An approach to performing the role of intentional mentor: I-Mentor with the Cycle of Caring** (Chapter 4, pp.51–3), **How to use the tool** (Chapter 6, p.73) and **Applications of the intentional mentor's toolkit** (Chapter 16, pp.139–178).

Index

This is an index to subjects. Only cited works from the Annotated Bibliography are indexed by their authors. Such authors are indicated by the prefix '*bib*'. A full list of citations is provided in the References section. Figures are indicated by the letter 'f'. Tables are indicated by the letter 't'.

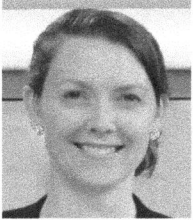

Dianne Salvador is a workplace trainer and assessor and a psychologist within medical education. Dianne designs learning experiences for junior doctors, runs medical education events, and teaches design, delivery and evaluation of junior doctor education and well-being initiatives. In 2011 Dianne co-founded The Townsville Hospital's Doctors for Doctors mentoring program with Dr Rachel Collings, to increase interns' access to individually-relevant assistance throughout internship.

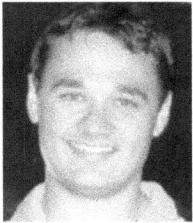

Dr Joel Wight is a senior haematology registrar from Queensland and currently resides in Melbourne, Australia. Joel is passionate about doctor development and has a special interest in medical culture. He has previously been a lead mentor of the Doctors for Doctors mentoring program and has been involved in physician education and educational policy development as chief medical registrar.

www.ingramcontent.com/pod-product-compliance
Lightning Source LLC
Chambersburg PA
CBHW061344210326
41598CB00035B/5874